KT-226-124

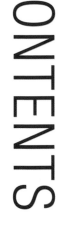

CONTENTS

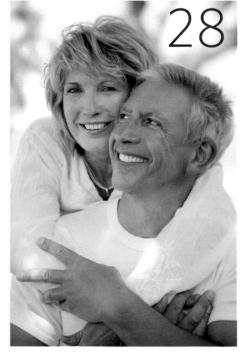

28

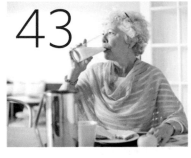

43

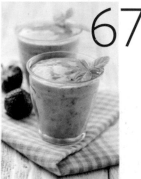

67

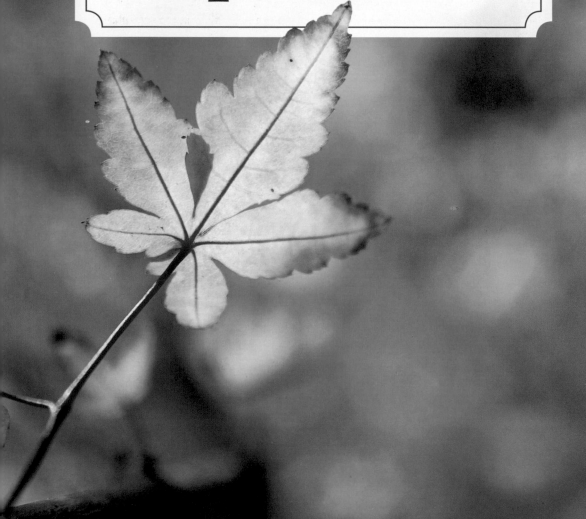

Preventing
AN
Epidemic

ALZHEIMER'S DISEASE. The mere mention of this phrase is enough to worry people. Many of us are intimately familiar with the devastating effects of this disease; of how it robs a person of his or her memory and how it deprives that person's friends and family of the once meaningful connection they shared with each other. It's a deadly disease that kills slowly, taking away segments of a person's life a little at a time.

With Alzheimer's disease, connections **between** brain cells – and the **brain cells themselves** – degenerate and die, causing the brain to shrink. The brain deterioration that takes place results in dementia – forgetfulness, loss of interest in usual activities, decline in intellectual and social skills as well as trouble controlling emotions. Eventually, those afflicted begin to disconnect from all that was once familiar to them, and advancing dementia causes their irrational and erratic behavior to escalate. By the time severe Alzheimer's sets in, the brain is so ravaged that patients can no longer physically function on their own and require constant care and assistance with the most basic of everyday tasks. It is a sad and difficult process to experience and observe.

The latest figures estimate that **5.2 million** Americans, nearly **500,000** people in the United Kingdom, and **320,000** Australians currently suffer from Alzheimer's. The worldwide total is nearing a staggering **36 million**. These numbers are rightfully cause for alarm.

Age is the **number one** risk factor for Alzheimer's. There is no cure yet for the disease, and current prescription medications used to treat Alzheimer's, such as Aricept and Exelon, only improve symptoms temporarily before becoming ineffective. The dramatic rise in life expectancy in much of the world has made Alzheimer's disease all too common in the 21st century. And with the Baby Boomer generation currently entering their retirement years, the instances of Alzheimer's are expected to rise even further.

These are overwhelming statistics confronting us, and they are only projected to increase over the next few decades. In fact, researchers predict that the total number of people living with Alzheimer's disease will triple, or quadruple, by 2050, causing an all-out Alzheimer's epidemic if a cure is not found.

What is being done to combat this crisis, and do we have a hand in our own fate when it comes to Alzheimer's?

The good news is that the causes, treatments, and potential cure for Alzheimer's disease are at the forefront of biomedical research. Doctors and scientists working with public and private universities and privately funded organizations, as well as through government initiatives, are making remarkable breakthroughs in understanding the disease.

The last decade has provided us with some of the most promising progress and innovation including:

- Connections being made between heart disease, type-2 diabetes, and Alzheimer's disease that could lead to preventative medication.
- Tests that predict risk factors for Alzheimer's, leading to improved diagnosis of the disease, and suggesting hope for prevention tactics.
- New FDA-approved drugs that detect brain abnormalities that lead to a more accurate diagnosis of the disease.
- A blood test currently in development that will allow doctors to predict the onset of Alzheimer's years before dementia symptoms set in.

While the scientific community is busy unraveling the mysteries of Alzheimer's, we as individuals can assume personal responsibility for our fate by taking the information from these latest findings and proactively incorporating lifestyle changes into our daily lives to stave off dementia.

Alzheimer's disease does not discriminate, and no aging adult is exempt. No one can prevent getting older,

but there are things we can do in order to reduce our risk of Alzheimer's. Paying better attention to our nutrition habits, minimizing our risk for lifestyle diseases such as heart disease and type-2 diabetes, as well as keeping our brains active through lifetime learning and regular social activity, are vital steps we can take to help stave off the disease and enhance our quality of life well into our golden years.

Personal methods of prevention in Part II of this book include:

- Advice on eating the right foods to maintain a healthy body weight, lower cholesterol, regulate blood glucose, lower blood pressure, and reduce inflammation.
- Physical fitness recommendations for aerobic exercise and strength training.
- Advice for managing stress, sleeping well, overcoming depression, and quitting smoking.
- Suggestions for improving brain health through mental stimulation, lifetime learning, and social engagement.

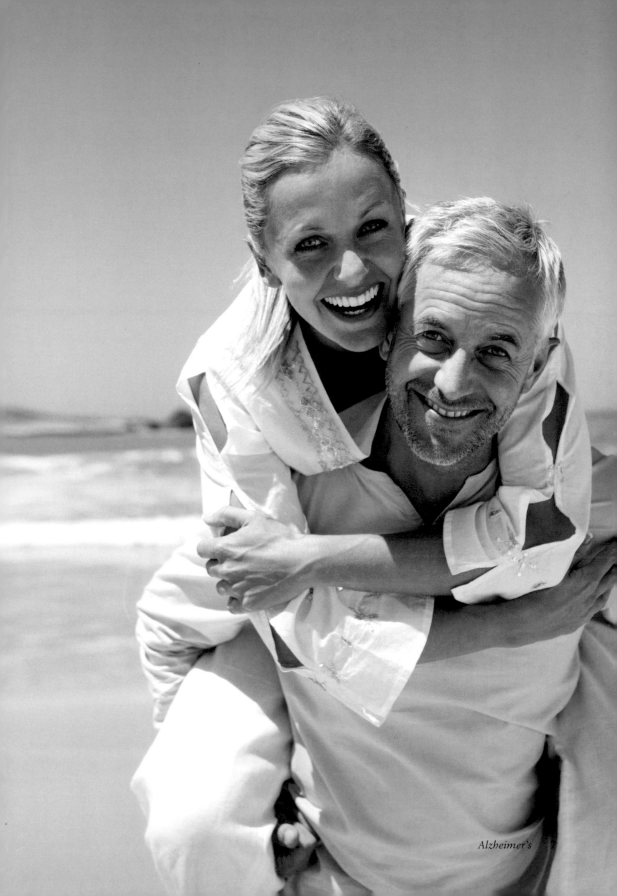

Alzheimer's

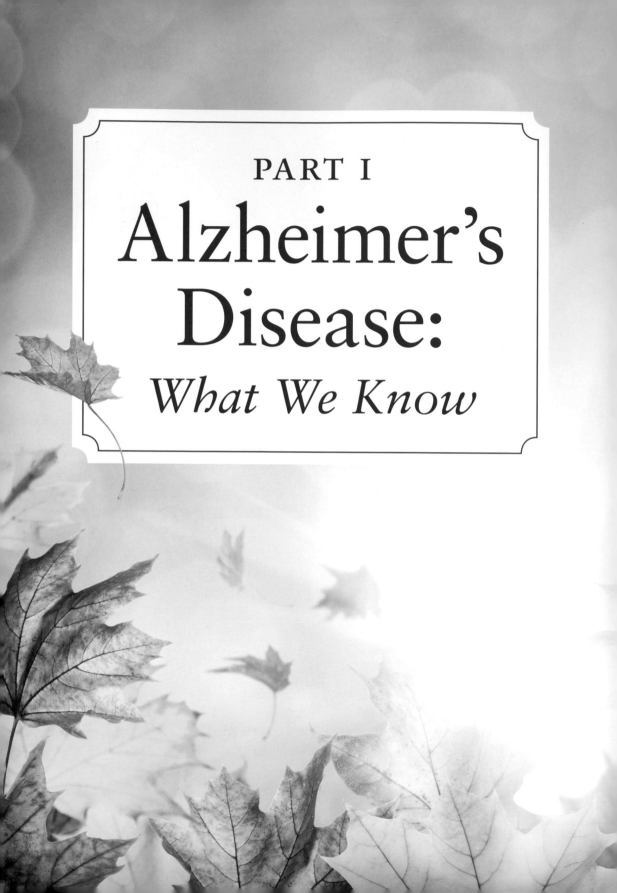

PART I
Alzheimer's Disease:
What We Know

ALZHEIMER'S FACTS AND FIGURES

- Alzheimer's disease is the leading cause of dementia in people over 65.
- Up to 5% of people with Alzheimer's are diagnosed as early as their 30s, 40s or 50s.
- A person's life expectancy upon diagnosis can range from four to 20 years, while average survival is eight years.
- The rate at which Alzheimer's symptoms worsen varies from person to person.
- The older a person is diagnosed with Alzheimer's, the shorter their life expectancy is.
- Dementia is the single greatest cause of disability in Australia.
- Alzheimer's is the 6th leading cause of death in the United States.
- Among the leading causes of death, Alzheimer's is the only one without a way to prevent, cure or even slow its progression.
- There are no Alzheimer's survivors. People with Alzheimer's either die from it or with it.

- One in three seniors in the United States dies with Alzheimer's or other dementia.
- Worldwide, approximately 36 million people are estimated to have Alzheimer's.
- Deaths from other major diseases, such as heart disease, HIV/AIDS, and stroke are in significant decline, while Alzheimer's deaths continue to rise.
- The number of worldwide cases is expected to triple over the next 40 years.

A DEFINITION

- **Degenerative**: Alzheimer's is a degenerative brain disease whose primary effect is irreversible dementia caused by brain atrophy.
- **Progressive**: The symptoms of Alzheimer's develop slowly and worsen over time as the brain continues to shrink.
- **Irreversible**: It is currently impossible to reverse the course of the disease.
- **Incurable**: There is no known cure for Alzheimer's, and its exact causes have not been identified.
- **Deadly**: Alzheimer's symptoms affect more than memory. Later stages of the disease lead to a loss of physical function resulting in death.

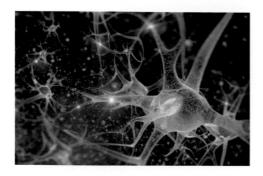

Alzheimer's disease causes nerve cell death and tissue loss throughout the brain. This brain *atrophy*, or shrinkage, causes dementia. Dementia occurs when *neurons* – nerve cells in the brain that transmit information through electrical and chemical signals – die and when *synapses* –the communication pathways between neurons – are lost. Such changes to the structure of the brain impact the brain's ability to carry out tasks.

As neurons and synapses continue to shut down, dementia worsens, affecting a person's memory, personality, behavior, and reasoning until they can no longer function independently. In addition to cognitive impairment due to dementia, a person will suffer physical immobility during the later stages of the disease because of advancing brain atrophy. During late-stage Alzheimer's, a patient will experience balance, walking and swallowing issues, among other physical complications. The cause of death is usually related to consequences of this immobility, such as falls, pneumonia, pressure sores or aspiration.

ALOIS ALZHEIMER

Alzheimer's disease was first described in 1906 by a German psychiatrist and neuropathologist named Alois Alzheimer.

Alzheimer spent several years studying Auguste Deter, a woman whose memory and cognitive abilities rapidly declined without explanation.

At age 51, she began experiencing memory lapses, disorientation and aphasia (the inability to use language).

Eventually, she lost the ability to care for herself and died at the age of 55.

After her death, Alzheimer studied her brain under a microscope and discovered the plaque deposits and tangles later to be identified as beta-amyloid and tau proteins.

It is a testament to the skill and determination of Dr. Alzheimer that more than 100 years ago he was able to determine the hallmarks of the disease, but that hundred-year span is equally telling of just how puzzling Alzheimer's disease has been for the scientific community .

DEMENTIA

The terms dementia and Alzheimer's disease are not interchangeable, but they are related. Dementia is not a disease, it is a *syndrome* – a group of related and concurrently occurring symptoms – that is the most prominent characteristic of Alzheimer's disease in its early and moderate stages. The symptoms of dementia consist of a pattern of cognitive deficits, including:

- Memory loss
- Slowed thinking speed
- Decreased mental agility
- Language problems
- Decreased comprehension
- Poor judgment

The severity of these symptoms in a person with Alzheimer's is great enough to impact his or her daily life.

The most common cause of dementia is Alzheimer's disease, followed by vascular dementia, which is caused by conditions such as multiple mild strokes that block or reduce blood flow to the brain. Vascular dementia and Alzheimer's disease can be difficult to distinguish because they present with nearly identical symptoms. One way to tell them apart is that Alzheimer's dementia develops gradually, whereas vascular dementia appears suddenly. It is not always easy for doctors and their patients to pinpoint exactly when symptoms began and whether those symptoms were sudden or gradual, so further testing is needed to rule out one or the other condition.

Depending on its cause, dementia can be reversible; however, symptoms caused by Alzheimer's disease are irreversible and guaranteed to worsen over time.

WHAT IS MILD COGNITIVE IMPAIRMENT (MCI)?

MCI is an intermediate stage of cognitive decline that falls somewhere between normal aging and full-fledged dementia. It may involve memory problems and mental decline, but its symptoms are not severe enough to interfere with daily life.

MCI shares similar risk factors with Alzheimer's disease, and people with MCI are at a greater risk for Alzheimer's, though it is not a guarantee that one will develop the disease. Some people with MCI never get worse, and some even get better.

Other Conditions That Can Present with Dementia

✔ Certain thyroid, kidney, or liver problems

✔ Drug interactions

✔ Medication side effects

✔ Vitamin deficiencies such as B12

✔ Brain tumors

✔ Infections in the brain

✔ Blood clots in the brain

✔ Alcohol Abuse

✔ Depression

THE ALZHEIMER'S BRAIN

The brain is made up of three distinct parts: **cerebrum, cerebellum**, and **brain stem**.

The *cerebrum* is the "wrinkly" part of the brain that fills up the majority of the skull, encompassing about two-thirds of brain mass. It handles memory, problem solving, intellectual function, emotion, and personality. It is divided into two hemispheres – the left brain and right brain – and is surrounded by an outer portion of grey matter called the *cerebral cortex*. Most of the information processing in the brain takes place in the cortex, which appears wrinkled because it consists of folds. These folds exist to increase the total surface area of the cortex, thereby increasing the amount of information that can be processed.

A NOTE ABOUT THE HIPPOCAMPUS

The *hippocampus* is located under the cerebral cortex. In Alzheimer's disease, the hippocampus is one of the first regions of the brain to suffer damage. Memory loss and disorientation are included among the early symptoms of damage to this area.

The *cerebellum* sits at the back of the head, underneath the cerebrum. It controls motor movement, coordination, balance, equilibrium, and muscle tone. The grey matter surrounding the cerebellum is called the *cerebellar cortex*.

The *brain stem* sits beneath the cerebrum and in front of the cerebellum. It connects the cerebrum to the spinal cord. The brain stem controls automatic functions such as breathing, digestion, heart rate, and blood pressure. It also relays information between the body and the upper parts of the brain.

The adult brain contains approximately 100 billion neurons with branches that connect at more than 100 trillion points. The connection point between neurons is called a synapse. When neurons communicate through electrical charges, they trigger the release of chemicals called *neurotransmitters*. Neurotransmitters travel across synapses to deliver the signals to other neurons.

In a person with Alzheimer's disease, these communication pathways, along with the cells themselves, are destroyed. Over time, nerve cell death and tissue loss lead to the brain atrophy and shrinkage that results in progressively worsening dementia and the loss of control over everyday functions.

In the Alzheimer's brain, plaques accumulate inside neurons, and tangles form outside neurons, causing them to malfunction and die. Both plaques and tangles occur due to abnormal protein formations.

Amyloid plaques – Plaques are the result of abnormal clusters of the protein fragment beta-amyloid. These clusters build up between nerve cells and block communication between cells at the synapse. Some scientists speculate that beta-amyloid plaques trigger an immune response that results in chronic inflammation, which devours cells.

These neuron-destroying deposits are the byproduct of *amyloid precursor protein*, or APP as it's commonly referred to. APP is necessary for brain development and repair. Once it is used, it is broken down into protein fragments called amino acids. A typical beta-amyloid protein is composed of a string of forty amino acids cut to a precise length. But if it is cut longer by two amino acids, it can congeal into plaques. As we age, more of these longer strings of beta-amyloid are found in the brain.

Neurofibrillary Tangles – Inside neurons, neurofibrillary tangles form when strands of the protein called *tau* twist together. Tau is essential for keeping communication pathways intact; however, in unhealthy parts of the brain, tau fibers twist to form tangles so that nutrients and other supplies cannot move through the cells. The deprived cells eventually die.

In the earliest stages of Alzheimer's disease, these plaques and tangles form in areas of the brain that control learning and memory, as well as thinking and planning. As the disease progresses, plaques and tangles continue to form in these areas and memory, thinking and planning problems worsen. In moderate stage Alzheimer's, plaques and tangles also begin to spread to parts of the brain that control speech and spatial relations.

By the time severe Alzheimer's has set in, most of the brain's cortex is damaged and the brain has shrunk dramatically to the point where patients can no longer care for themselves, communicate effectively, or recognize friends and family.

The question whose answer still eludes scientists is whether or not plaques and tangles are the root causes of Alzheimer's disease, or if plaques and tangles are disease markers whose root cause has yet to be discovered.

There are competing theories of causation. Researchers who believe amyloid plaques are the root cause of Alzheimer's are called "baptists," while researchers who believe that tau protein is to blame are called "tauists." But in addition to these two major theories, researchers are also exploring other avenues of causation, namely *free-radicals* and *inflammation*.

Free-radicals are highly reactive atoms or groups of atoms with an odd (unpaired) number of electrons. When free-radicals form, they can start a chain reaction in cellular components like DNA or the cell membrane, resulting in *oxidative stress* that causes cells to malfunction and die. Research suggests that this oxidative stress is what leads to the formation of beta-amyloid plaques in neurons.

Inflammation is the body's attempt to rid itself of harmful stimuli. It is an essential immune response that counteracts physical, chemical, or biological agents that traumatize the body. Inflammation can be beneficial, as in the case of the bump or bruise that appears after physical trauma, for example. That bruise and swelling are due to an increase in blood flow that supplies the oxygen and nutrients necessary for healing the wounded area.

BRAIN SCAN MAY DIAGNOSE ALZHEIMER'S BRAIN CHANGES AS THEY OCCUR

Japanese researchers have devised a new imaging technique to detect physical changes as they occur in the brains of Alzheimer's patients. A team led by Dr. Makoto Higuchi at the National Institute of Radiological Sciences outside of Tokyo is testing imaging technology that binds fluorescent compounds to tau proteins that can then be picked up on a PET scan. If scans can successfully and accurately track the progression of tau proteins, doctors might then be able to diagnose the disease at a much earlier stage and monitor the effectiveness of medications with subsequent scans.

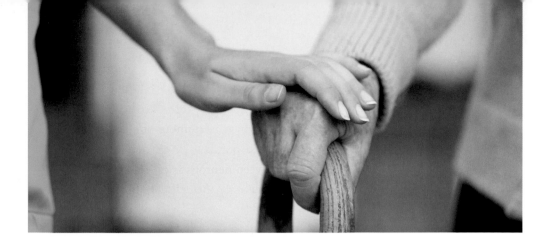

Pain, redness, heat, and swelling are hallmarks of *acute* inflammation.

Inflammation isn't always visible to the naked eye. Often, inflammation responses are triggered internally within organs, tissues, and joints. Acute inflammation takes place with conditions such as bronchitis, appendicitis, tonsillitis, and flu. When these conditions are treated and cured, the symptoms of acute inflammation disappear.

But inflammation can be harmful as well. When the body triggers an immune response, inflammation can become self-perpetuating. In other words, the body begins responding to the inflammation as its own negative stimulus by continually creating more inflammation to combat it. This is referred to as *chronic* inflammation and can last for months or even years. Chronic inflammation can result in diseases like rheumatoid arthritis and atherosclerosis. It is this chronic type of inflammation that interests Alzheimer's researchers.

THE STAGES OF ALZHEIMER'S DISEASE

Alzheimer's disease can be broken down into three major stages – an early, pre-clinical stage with no symptoms, a middle stage that involves mild to moderate cognitive impairment, and a final stage of severe dementia and physical immobility. Early-stage Alzheimer's effects on the brain may begin 20 years or more before diagnosis. Mild to moderate Alzheimer's generally lasts between two and 10 years. And severe, final stage Alzheimer's typically lasts from one to five years.

According to the US-based Alzheimer's Association, these three stages can be further broken down into seven. Often, symptoms associated with a particular stage overlap with those of a preceding or successive stage.

STAGE 1

NO IMPAIRMENT (NORMAL FUNCTION)

There is no evidence of dementia in the person, and he or she does not experience any memory problems. This can also be referred to as the *asymptomatic* phase for the purposes of research.

STAGE 2

VERY MILD DECLINE

The person may be experiencing normal age-related cognitive changes or the earliest signs of Alzheimer's disease, however, signs of dementia cannot be detected by friends, family or medical examination.

STAGE 3

MILD DECLINE

Early-stage Alzheimer's can be diagnosed in some individuals at this point. Friends, family, and coworkers might begin to notice memory or concentration problems. People with mild cognitive decline might have trouble completing tasks in social or work situations; they might have trouble remembering words or names; and they might have trouble staying organized.

STAGE 4

MODERATE DECLINE

A doctor can detect clear-cut symptoms of early-stage dementia at this point. Medical interviews might reveal an impaired ability to do challenging mental arithmetic. Patients might exhibit moodiness or withdraw from socially or mentally challenging situations. They might become more forgetful and have difficulty performing complex tasks such as balancing a checkbook or remembering driving directions.

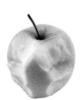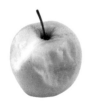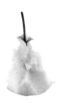

STAGE 5

MODERATELY SEVERE DECLINE

People with moderate or mid-stage Alzheimer's begin to need help with daily activities. They may forget their address or telephone number and become confused about what day it is or where they are. They may begin to make inappropriate choices about what to wear with regard to the weather or social occasion; however, at this stage they still remember significant details about themselves and their family and they do not require assistance eating or using the bathroom.

STAGE 6

SEVERE DECLINE

At this point patients require extensive assistance with daily activities. Memory continues to decline, and patients can lose awareness of recent experiences as well as of their surroundings. Without supervision, they will make mistakes in dressing, such as putting their shoes on the wrong feet. They will have increasing trouble using the bathroom and controlling their bladder and bowel. Patients may also experience major personality and behavioral changes as well as changes in sleep patterns. They will also have a tendency to wander and get lost.

STAGE 7

VERY SEVERE DECLINE

Severe or late-stage Alzheimer's is the final stage of the disease. Patients at this stage need help with their daily personal care, including eating or using the bathroom. They may also experience *apraxia* – the inability to control movement, including the inability to smile, sit without support, or hold their head up without assistance. They might also experience *aphasia*, which affects speech. They may not be able to carry on a conversation, though they may still say words or phrases.

* This seven-stage framework is based on a system developed by Barry Reisberg, M.D., clinical director of the New York University School of Medicine's Silberstein Aging and Dementia Research Center.

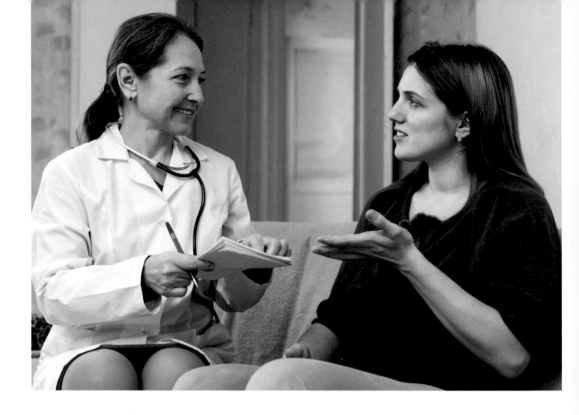

EARLY ONSET ALZHEIMER'S

Early-onset Alzheimer's (also known as younger-onset) is a form of the disease that affects people under the age of 65. The majority of people with early onset are in their 40s or 50s, but it can affect people in their 20s and 30s as well.

Early-onset Alzheimer's presents with the same symptoms and progresses the same way as it does for people over 65. It can be difficult to diagnose due to the fact that doctors don't often look for Alzheimer's in people under 65 to determine the cause of their memory problems, thus symptoms may be incorrectly attributed to stress or other lifestyle factors.

Once early-onset Alzheimer's is diagnosed, younger patients are treated with the same medications as those over 65 who are diagnosed with late-onset Alzheimer's – the most common form of the disease.

* **Take Note:** Early-onset Alzheimer's is not the same as early-stage Alzheimer's. *Early-onset* refers to Alzheimer's that is diagnosed in a person before age 65. *Early-stage* Alzheimer's refers to the circumstances and symptoms that are associated with the beginning phases of Alzheimer's disease

RISK FACTORS FOR ALZHEIMER'S DISEASE

- **Age**: A person's age is the greatest risk factor for developing Alzheimer's. People are living longer, and if population trends continue in this direction, the number of people with Alzheimer's will increase. A person's risk for developing Alzheimer's-related dementia doubles for each five year interval over age 65.

- **Family History**: If a first-degree relative – a parent or sibling – has the disease, a person's risk is slightly higher than that of the average population.

- **Genetics**: There are three genes with mutations found to cause an inherited form of Alzheimer's: Amyloid precursor protein (APP), Presenilin-1 (PS-1), and Presenilin-2 (PS-2). A fourth gene, apolipoprotein E (APOE), provides instructions for making the protein that clears beta-amyloid from the brain, and has proved the most promising in terms of findings. The $APOE_4$ form of this gene increases the likelihood for developing Alzheimer's in people who inherit it, but it is not a guarantee that they will develop the disease.

- **Gender**: Women are more likely than men to develop Alzheimer's. Initially, this was thought to be the case because women outlive men by an average of four years. But more recent studies suggest that changes in the brain that occur after menopause may be the more accurate explanation.

- **Previous Brain Trauma**: People who have had severe or repeated head trauma, especially when the trauma results in unconsciousness, appear to have a greater risk for Alzheimer's. For example, professional athletes such as NFL players who sustain repeated concussive blows have died from Alzheimer's disease at a rate four times higher than that of the general population.

- **Lifestyle Factors**: While there is no conclusive evidence that these factors cause Alzheimer's, studies suggest that they may contribute to its development: sedentary lifestyle, high blood pressure, high cholesterol, type-2 diabetes, inadequate consumption of fruits and vegetables, smoking, and minimal social engagement.

ALZHEIMER'S AND DEMENTIA WARNING SIGNS: WHEN TO CALL A DOCTOR

You may have heard stories of a friend's mother or grandfather leaving the house clothed only in a bathrobe and slippers, wandering off into the neighborhood lost and confused, and then brought home to a concerned and thankful caregiver. Or you may have experienced firsthand the wrenching feeling of looking into a loved one's eyes and realizing that they no longer recognize you. These realities are examples of the devastation that Alzheimer's disease can inflict not only on patients but also on the loved ones who witness their decline and care for them when they can no longer care for themselves.

These are common examples of moderate and late stage Alzheimer's that we most easily associate with the disease. But how do we discern early, pre-diagnosis dementia symptoms from ordinary forgetfulness?

All of us can be forgetful at times – misplacing car keys, missing an appointment, or forgetting a person's name whom we've only met briefly. It's natural to be distracted or stressed by the pace of our daily lives or to be experiencing normal age-related memory changes. But in a person with dementia, such situations occur frequently and adversely interfere with daily tasks and interactions, and can even put personal safety at risk. The following are warning signs that someone's forgetfulness and uncharacteristic behavior are serious enough to warrant a visit to the doctor.

- **Memory Loss**: Frequent inability to recall recent events or important dates and appointments; inability to recognize or remember the names of friends and family.
- **Repetition**: Asking the same question repeatedly even though it may have been answered; telling the same story, often verbatim, as if it is playing on a loop.
- **Language Problems**: Also called aphasia. Changes in speech; problems remembering basic words; inability to hold a coherent conversation; struggling to remember the names of everyday objects; mumbling or speaking in gibberish.
- **Visual Perception Problems**: Trouble judging distances or determining the height of a stair or a curb; seeing one's reflection in a mirror and thinking there is someone else in the room.
- **Personality Changes**: Mood swings

from happy to sad to distraught or defensive; sudden, unexplained bouts of irritability, anger, or suspiciousness; abandonment of favorite activities and withdrawal from social interaction.

- **Disorientation and Confusion**: Wandering off and getting lost in a familiar environment, such as in their own neighborhood or while driving to a familiar location; forgetting how to execute basic tasks, such as using the stove or getting dressed; forgetting the intended function of common items like a stove or a comb.

- **Odd Behavior**: Illogical execution of tasks, such as placing the toothbrush in the refrigerator or the milk in the pantry drawer; trusting strangers while mistrusting family and friends.

- **Poor Hygiene**: Infrequent bathing; wearing stained or soiled clothing; wearing the same clothing and/or undergarments several days in a row; unkempt appearance such as uncombed hair or disheveled attire.

People with dementia might not recognize that these symptoms are occurring, so friends and loved ones must pay attention to any changes in their behavior and take note of anything abnormal. Keep in mind, such behavior does not necessarily indicate Alzheimer's; however, it is important not to ignore potential warning signs and to schedule an evaluation with a physician to find out what, if anything, is going on.

NEW TEST SUGGESTS THAT INABILITY TO RECOGNIZE FAMOUS FACES MAY BE A SIGN OF EARLY-ONSET DEMENTIA

Researchers tested 30 people with primary progressive aphasia (PPA), a rare kind of early-onset dementia, and 27 people without dementia who acted as controls to see how many famous faces they were able to recognize.

A team from the Cognitive Neurology and Alzheimer's Disease Center at the Northwestern University Feinberg School of Medicine in Chicago, IL devised a test that showed participants black and white images of well-known figures including President John F. Kennedy, Princess Diana, Pope John Paul II, and Elvis Presley. Participants were given a point for each person they were able to name. For faces they couldn't name, they were given a point if they were able to describe at least two accurate facts about the person in the picture.

The people with PPA scored consistently worse than those without dementia, but researchers have more work to do before they can conclude that the test distinguishes all people with dementia, including Alzheimer's disease, or only those with the more rare PPA form.

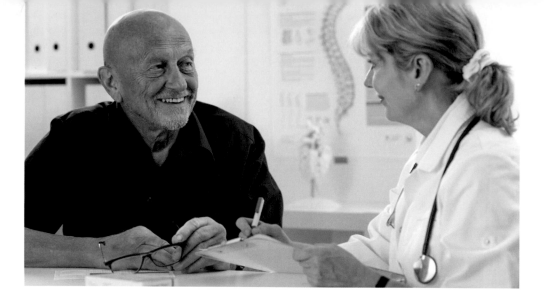

DIAGNOSIS

While the symptoms of dementia are relatively easy to spot, it is impossible for doctors to arrive at an absolute diagnosis of Alzheimer's while a patient is alive. Confirmation of the disease can only be obtained after death by examining brain tissue during autopsy.

Although diagnosis during an individual's lifetime is tricky, doctors can pinpoint Alzheimer's disease as the probable cause of dementia through a series of exams. A good doctor will employ a combination of these exams to ensure the most accurate diagnosis. One test on its own is not enough.

- Brain imaging to rule out and identify other medical problems – CT (computed tomography) scans, PET (positron emission tomography) scans, and MRIs (magnetic resonance imaging), can expose visible abnormalities related to conditions other than Alzheimer's that cause dementia, such as strokes and tumors.
- Minimal Mental State Exam (MMSE) – The MMSE is the most commonly used test to assess memory problems. Doctors ask a series of questions that help to diagnose dementia and determine its progression. Short-form testing takes around ten minutes.
- Longer-form neuropsychological testing may be used to provide additional details about mental function if doctors suspect the early stages of Alzheimer's or other dementia.
- Neurological exams to test speech, balance, coordination, and reflexes.
- Physiological exams to assess muscle tone and strength as well as to test sight and hearing.

The Benefit of Early Diagnosis

Even though there is currently no cure for Alzheimer's, it is important not to give up before even receiving a diagnosis and knowing your options. Seeing your doctor as soon as you suspect symptoms of dementia can help you determine conditions other than Alzheimer's that might be causing your cognitive impairment. If you do have Alzheimer's, finding out early means that the current available drug treatments have a greater chance of being effective in temporarily improving your symptoms. You might also be eligible to participate in clinical trials, one of which might unlock the door to improved treatment of the disease or even a cure.

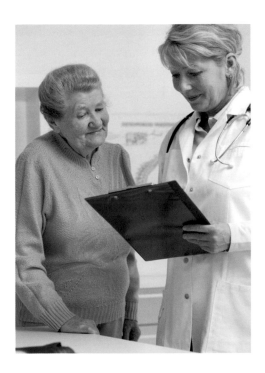

FDA APPROVES TWO DRUGS FOR ADVANCED BRAIN IMAGING

In October 2013, The U.S. Food and Drug Administration (FDA) approved the drug **Vizamil,** created by GE Healthcare, for use in radioactive imaging that assists in Alzheimer's diagnosis. Vizamil works by binding to beta-amyloid protein build-up in the brain. It is injected in the patient before a PET scan is performed and highlights the abnormal plaque in the scans. A negative scan means that little plaque has been found and that Alzheimer's is not the likely cause of a patient's dementia symptoms.

The drug **florbetapir (Amyvid),** created by Eli Lilly & Co., was approved by the FDA in April 2013 as the first radioactive dye to locate beta-amyloid plaques in PET scans.

Both drugs are meant to be used in combination with other physical and mental exams in the diagnosis of patients being evaluated for Alzheimer's disease. PET scans alone cannot confirm the disease's presence in the brain, and doctors are careful to emphasize that positive scans indicate a likelihood not a confirmation of the disease.

THE PEANUT BUTTER TEST

A pilot study published in the *Journal of the Neurological Sciences* produced results indicating that a person's inability to smell peanut butter may be a sign of Alzheimer's disease. Researchers at the University of Florida's McKnight Brain Institute Center for Smell and Taste say that preliminary results are promising and that the peanut butter test could prove a cheap and effective way to diagnose Alzheimer's at an earlier stage than currently possible.

The study findings indicate that patients with early-stage Alzheimer's disease had more difficulty smelling peanut butter held at short distances from their nose than people without the disease. Graduate student Jennifer Stamps devised the test when she noticed that patients had not been tested for their sense of smell, pointing out that the olfactory nerve (instrumental to the sense of smell) is one of the first things to be affected in cognitive decline, even before memory loss.

Much more testing needs to be done before the peanut butter test can be confirmed as a diagnostic tool, so please do not pull peanut butter jars out of the pantry to self-diagnose!

CURRENT DRUG TREATMENTS

Doctors and researchers have yet to find a cure for Alzheimer's, but the disease is treatable in some patients. Prescription drugs can help to lessen or stabilize the symptoms of Alzheimer's – but only for a limited time. Eventually, medication is no longer an effective treatment, and patients begin a decline into more severe stages of dementia. There are no drug treatments available to stave off the physical symptoms associated with late-stage Alzheimer's disease.

Currently there are two types of drugs used to treat the cognitive symptoms of Alzheimer's. The first is a class of drugs called **cholinesterase inhibitors,** which are used during the early to moderate stages of the disease. Cholinesterase inhibitors are used to treat symptoms related to memory, thinking, language, and judgment by increasing levels of the neurotransmitter *acetylcholine*. In most cases, they are effective for six to twelve months.

Cholinesterase inhibitors include:

✔ **Donepezil**

   (proprietary name Aricept)
   * Donezipil can be used during all stages of dementia, from early to severe.

✔ **Rivastigmine**

   (proprietary name Excelon)

✔ **Galantamine**

   (proprietary name Razadyne in the US, Reminyl in the UK and Australia)

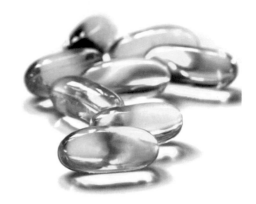

The second type of drug is **memantine** (proprietary name Namenda in the US, Ebixa in the UK and Australia), which belongs to a class of drugs called **NMDA receptor antagonists**. Memantine can either be prescribed alone or used in tandem with the cholinesterase inhibitor donepezil for patients with moderate to severe dementia. It can help people with Alzheimer's disease to think more clearly and perform daily activities more easily by preventing the overproduction of a brain chemical called *glutamate*. Too much glutamate results in the damage and destruction of brain cells. But, like cholinesterase inhibitors, memantine does not stop or reverse the progression of Alzheimer's.

Vitamin E – Doctors will sometimes prescribe vitamin E to treat the cognitive symptoms of Alzheimer's disease. Vitamin E is an antioxidant that is thought to protect brain cells and cells throughout the body from deterioration. Vitamin E should only be taken under the supervision of a physician as high doses can negatively interact with other medications and might increase the risk of death in certain patients. If you suspect that you or a loved one has dementia, do not self-medicate with vitamin E. Instead, consult with a physician about your condition as soon as possible.

Other Medications – Various anti-anxiety medications, antidepressants, antipsychotics, or sleep aids may be prescribed to help a patient deal with the psychological and behavioral symptoms associated with dementia.

A Word of Caution – Do not be tempted by drugs and treatments promising a "cure" for Alzheimer's disease. No such drugs or treatments exist. And while they might claim that they contain no harmful side effects and can therefore be administered guilt-free, in reality, they are at best a waste of money and at worst unsafe for consumption. They could also adversely interact with other medications you take. Always consult with your physician before taking any pills or treatments, whether they are for Alzheimer's or other ailments, to ensure your safety.

HOPE FOR THE FUTURE

The medical community is making continuous efforts to further understand the human body. Scientists conduct research and testing in pursuit of discoveries that will enable people to live longer and healthier lives. Through trial and error, they are unearthing clues about the origins of Alzheimer's disease and how to diagnose and treat it, but it has not been a straightforward or simple process – competing theories, failed medications, and other setbacks are common. Such complications are what drive scientists to keep exploring and to keep asking questions. And while all this investigative progress is reassuring, it can also be confusing for consumers to determine

what is crucial for them to know.

The important thing to keep in mind is that scientific discovery is a process, and that whether new information goes on to become validated or disproved, it is all helpful in the pursuit of further knowledge and understanding of the disease.

Epidemiological Studies:
Epidemiology is the study of the patterns, causes, and effects of health and disease conditions in defined populations. A defined population can be an ethnic group, age group or any group that shares a common characteristic relevant to the disease being studied. Epidemiological studies can identify risk factors for a particular disease and present targets for preventive medicine or other preventive tactics. They can also compare the treatment effects of clinical trials, which are drug studies.

In an epidemiological study, people are observed over a set period of time as they go about their daily lives. The recorded data is then analyzed for which behaviors or environmental factors may be linked to a disease. The studies do not offer absolute confirmation that these factors cause or prevent the disease or health condition, but scientists can report whether or not a finding "is associated with" a particular disease such as Alzheimer's. At that point, preventative measures or initiatives for drug interventions might be recommended.

Examples of epidemiological studies are the Dementia Risk Factor test and the Alzheimer's Disease Neuroimaging Initiative, which are both discussed in the following pages.

Other types of studies include: **in vitro (test tube) studies**, which are biological studies conducted in test tubes (also referred to as "under glass") rather than in a human or animal, and **animal studies**, which involve the use of non-human animals in experiments. Both of these types of studies show a cause-and-effect relationship that may or may not be the same in humans.

Clinical trials, which are drug studies, are discussed throughout this section.

The Case for Prevention

A person will only develop noticeable signs of dementia when too much damage has already been done to the brain for it to be halted or reversed. This is the nature of degenerative brain disease. In the case of Alzheimer's, symptoms will only appear after one-third of the neurons in the brain have been damaged or destroyed by plaques, tangles, inflammation, and free-radicals.

No experimental treatments have yet been successful in halting or reversing the damage to the brain caused by Alzheimer's, so the case can be made for prevention being our best hope to end the disease. As more information is uncovered about when the Alzheimer's disease process begins, a shift can take place from today's symptomatic treatments – drugs like Aricept and Exelon that temporarily treat dementia symptoms – to *asymptomatic* treatments that are able to address the root causes of the disease in its infancy, years or even decades before symptoms ever manifest.

The question is, just what are the root causes of Alzheimer's disease? Beta-amyloid plaques and tau tangles have been at the forefront of research, but more recently new theories have developed that point to biomarkers, genetic roots, and lifestyle factors that may bring us closer to the truth about the origins of the disease that lead to those neuron-killing plaques and tangles.

Biomarkers (short for "biological markers") offer one of the most promising paths to early detection because they can predict and indicate a disease process. Currently, there are no validated biomarkers for Alzheimer's disease, but researchers are investigating encouraging possibilities such as: proteins in blood or spinal fluid, genetic mutations, and brain changes detectable by imaging like MRIs and PET scans.

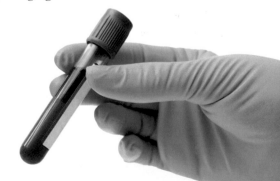

- **Brain Imaging**: Also called neuroimaging, brain imaging is already part of the standard workup for Alzheimer's disease. Doctors use MRI, PET, and CT scans to rule out other possible causes of dementia and determine the proper course of treatment. But scientists are also working toward making it possible for neuroimaging to play a key role in early detection by measuring early shrinkage of the hippocampus, detecting reduced brain cell activity, and diagnosing Alzheimer's at the molecular level, years before symptoms appear.

- **Cerebrospinal Fluid (CSF)**: CSF bathes the brain and spinal cord and acts as a buffer for the cortex, providing immunological protection inside the skull. Studies suggest that in its earliest stages, Alzheimer's disease may cause changes to CSF that affect levels of beta-amyloid and tau proteins. Researchers at Washington University School of Medicine's Knight Alzheimer's Disease Research Center in St. Louis, Missouri have been studying CSF as a biomarker for Alzheimer's. They compared MRI brain scans with *lumbar punctures** and found that in patients with early Alzheimer's, disruptions in brain pathways

emerged at around the same time as chemical markers for the disease appeared in spinal fluid. This research indicates that even though individuals might appear cognitively normal, doctors may be able to see changes in their brain very early on in the disease, which could lead to earlier diagnosis and better drug therapies.

* Commonly known as a spinal tap, a lumbar puncture is a medical procedure that extracts CSF from the spine.

- **Blood and Other Bodily Proteins**: Proteins are worker molecules necessary for virtually every activity in the body. They are formed by even smaller molecules called amino acids. Errors in these amino acids can cause disease. Researchers are investigating whether asymptomatic (pre-clinical) Alzheimer's causes consistent, measurable changes in blood and urine levels of beta-amyloid and tau proteins, or other biomarkers. Scientists are also exploring whether early Alzheimer's leads to such changes in other parts of the body.

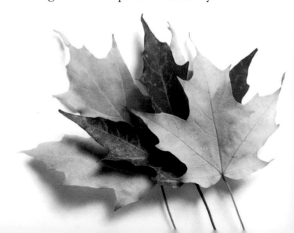

Genetic Risk Factors are variants in a cell's DNA that do not cause disease by themselves but may increase the chance that a person will develop a disease.

The most well-studied risk-factor gene is appolipoprotein E, commonly referred to as APOE. APOE has three forms: ε2, ε3, and ε4. Of these, $APOE_4$ (also written as APOEε4 or $ApoE_4$) has been found to increase a person's risk for Alzheimer's disease. People with the most significant risk are those who inherit $APOE_4$ from both parents, although people without this inherited risk factor can still develop the disease.

APOE produces a protein that absorbs beta-amyloid and clears it from the brain; however, the E_4 variant tends not to clear beta-amyloid sufficiently, which leads to plaque formations in some cases. Researchers at Columbia University in New York City now believe that they have discovered molecular pathways inside brain cells that appear to be altered by the presence of $APOE_4$. These brain pathways could help to explain why some carriers of $APOE_4$ go on to develop Alzheimer's while others do not, which in turn could lead to potential new drug targets for the disease.

Lifestyle Factors – Links to Other Diseases

A number of studies have linked Alzheimer's disease to lifestyle diseases such as heart disease, type-2 diabetes, and metabolic syndrome. It is these connections that offer us our most immediate hope for prevention through delay. If we can make more informed lifestyle choices based on the findings of these studies, then there may be hope for delaying the onset of dementia, perhaps indefinitely.

Heart Disease

Heart disease, also called cardiovascular disease, is an umbrella term used to describe several conditions that affect the heart, many of which are related to atherosclerosis. The heart is a muscle that pumps blood throughout the body. Atherosclerosis occurs when plaque builds up in arterial walls (arteries are blood vessels that convey blood from the heart to other parts of the body) thereby narrowing the arteries, making it harder for blood to pass through. If a blood clot forms, it can stop the blood flow altogether and result in heart attack or stroke.

A discovery made over 20 years ago by Larry Sparks, who at the time was a medical examiner in Kentucky, suggested that heart disease could be a precursor to brain disease. Sparks, who is now a scientist with Sun Health Research Institute in Arizona, was checking brain tissue for early signs of Alzheimer's disease when he noticed that all of the specimens that had amyloid plaques were from the brains of people who also had heart disease.

None of the samples from people without heart disease had signs of Alzheimer's.

A series of studies has correlated the risk factors for heart disease with a greater risk for Alzheimer's. For instance, one study showed that people with high cholesterol are three to five times more likely to develop Alzheimer's. Excess cholesterol in the blood results in excess cholesterol production in the brain, which leads to a buildup of plaques. High blood pressure also contributes to an increase in likelihood for Alzheimer's because it damages the blood vessels, leading to a decrease in nutrients that feed neurons. And smoking can double or triple a person's risk for dementia.

The good news is that these are the kinds of risk factors that can be modified by lifestyle changes.

Risk Factor Test Highlights Heart Health Factors Among Several Others as Risk for Late-Onset Alzheimer's

At the 10th International Conference on Alzheimer's Disease and Related Disorders (ICAD), held in Madrid, Spain, Swedish researchers unveiled a dementia risk test for middle-aged adults. The test was developed by a team at the Karolinska Institute's Aging Research Center in Stockholm.

The researchers devised a simple way to calculate a middle-aged patient's eventual dementia risk on a scale of 0-15. The score was developed by following 1,409 patients in the Cardiovascular Risk Factors, Aging, and Dementia (CAIDE) project. Participants were first examined in middle age (ages ranged from 39 to 64, and the average age was 50) and were re-examined 20 years later to assess dementia.

Seven risk factors became the criteria for the Dementia Risk Score.

1. Age
2. Sex
3. Years of Education
4. Body Mass Index (BMI)/Obesity
5. Blood Pressure
6. Cholesterol Level
7. Physical Activity Level

Risk scores were based on a snapshot of the health of the participants without treating them to control cholesterol levels or blood pressure, or advocating a change in lifestyle habits to increase activity in the intervening years between the first and second examinations.

The findings based on the CAIDE study subjects resulted in the following score and risk correlations:

SCORE	RISK	PERCENTAGE OF SUBJECTS WHO DEVELOPED DEMENTIA
0-5	Very Low	1%
6-7	Low	1.9%
8-9	Moderate	4.2%
10-11	High	7.4%
12-15	Very High	16.4%

Based on these findings, the Swedish research team identified modifiable risk factors for patients who can benefit from lifestyle changes and drug interventions to control cholesterol and high blood pressure before dementia sets in. Ultimately, the team determined that what is good for your heart is also good for your brain.

* Note that the team was not able to account for all possible risk factors, such as family history of dementia or diabetes, and emphasized the need for their inclusion in future studies.

Type-2 Diabetes

Type-1 diabetes is an immune disorder in which a person's body struggles to produce insulin, requiring the patient to administer daily insulin therapy in the form of injections or a pump to regulate blood sugar and stay alive. Unlike type-1 patients, people with type-2 diabetes produce insulin; however, when the insulin isn't used as it should be, glucose cannot enter the body's cells and the cells malfunction as a result. The unused insulin then builds up in the blood supply and can cause serious health complications such as fatigue, headache, blurred vision, dehydration, and diabetic coma. Pre-diabetes and type-2 diabetes also set the stage for arteriosclerosis (hardening/narrowing of the arteries) and cardiovascular disease.

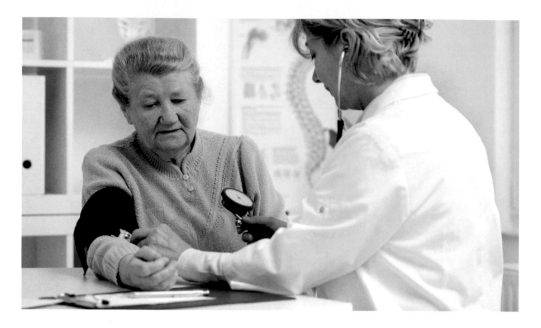

Anyone can develop type-2 diabetes, however the people at highest risk are overweight, obese or have metabolic syndrome. There is no medication or procedure that can cure type-2 diabetes, but if people make good diet and exercise choices and maintain healthy weight, they can lower their chances of developing the disease or, if they already have type-2 diabetes, can reduce their risk for complications.

Risk Factor Test Shows Link between Type-2 Diabetes and Alzheimer's

Statistics show that patients with type-2 diabetes are twice as likely to develop dementia as those without the disease. But until recently, it has not been possible to predict exactly which patients have the highest individualized risk.

In August 2013, a team of researchers from Keiser Permanente and the University Medical Center Utrecht in California presented the findings of the risk factor test they developed. The Diabetes-Specific Dementia Risk Score, as it is called, determines a risk score that provides an estimate of the 10-year individualized dementia risk for people with type-2 diabetes. The risk score is based primarily on a patient's medical history and can be easily calculated during a routine medical exam or through a patient's electronic medical records.

Scientists analyzed the medical records of 27,512 Californians with type-2 diabetes, aged 60 and over, and recorded whether or not the patients were diagnosed with dementia within ten years of their participation in the study. Nearly one in five, or 17 percent, of the participants developed dementia during this period.

Forty-five total possible risk factors were identified and used to establish the patient's risk factor score. Among those, six diabetes-related risk factors emerged as the most compelling health complications.

1. Acute metabolic event, such as a sever hypoglycemic or hyperglycemic event
2. Microvascular disease – a disease of the smaller blood vessels
3. Cerebrovascular disease – damage to the blood vessels supplying blood to the brain
4. Diabetic foot
5. Heart disease
6. Depression

Total scores were grouped into 14 categorics from lowest (0 points) to highest (20 points). Patients who scored highest were deemed a staggering 37 times more likely to develop dementia than those with the lowest scores. Broken down by percentage, patients in the lowest category of the 20-point risk score had a 5.3 percent chance of developing dementia, while those in the highest category had a 73 percent chance of developing the disease.

The findings of the Diabetes-Specific Dementia Risk Score study highlight a strong correlation between type-2 diabetes and dementia and stress the need for early intervention in the course of the disease, which includes mitigating the risk factors for developing type-2 diabetes.

COULD ALZHEIMER'S BE A FORM OF DIABETES?

According to neuropathologist Suzanne M. de la Monte, M.D. of Brown University in Rhode Island, she and her research team believe that Alzheimer's disease might be what they have dubbed "type-3 diabetes." De la Monte defines type-3 diabetes as an insulin resistance of the brain in which the brain's ability to use glucose and produce energy is impaired. In healthy brains, insulin produces the neurotransmitter *acetylcholine*. A lack of acetylcholine is a key marker of Alzheimer's.

Dr. de la Monte examined the brains of 45 deceased elderly Alzheimer's patients and found that among those who were in the most advanced stages of the disease, insulin receptors were nearly 80 percent lower than in a normal brain.

More studies could lead to proof that "type-3 diabetes" is one of several root causes of Alzheimer's.

Metabolic Syndrome

Metabolic syndrome (sometimes referred to as insulin resistance syndrome, although insulin resistance is not its only cause) is a group of conditions that puts people at risk for heart disease and diabetes. To be diagnosed with metabolic syndrome, a patient has to present with at least three of the following risk factors:

1. High blood pressure
2. High blood glucose (blood sugar)
3. High triglycerides (a type of blood fat)
4. Low levels of HDL (good cholesterol)
5. Obesity, especially fat around the waist

Because metabolic syndrome sets the stage for serious chronic health problems like heart disease and diabetes, its diagnosis is a wake-up call to make the lifestyle changes necessary to reverse its course.

A Sense of Urgency Leads to Major Initiatives

Evidence is mounting that Alzheimer's damages the brain well before dementia can be confirmed, therefore doctors are in search of the means and methods to identify this asymptomatic stage. To this end, several studies and initiatives are underway that could lead to early interventions that might slow the disease or stop it in its tracks. If drugs can be administered much sooner in the course of the disease, tailored to specific biomarkers, there could be hope for prevention.

Prevention and Early Detection Studies and Data Initiatives
BRAIN Initiative

In April 2013, US President Barrack Obama announced his support for the Brain Research though Advancing Innovative Neurotechnologies (BRAIN) Initiative, whose purpose is to uncover how the brain functions both in health and disease – an understanding that has eluded scientists despite the many advancements in neuroscience in recent years.

The initiative, helmed by the National Institutes of Health (NIH), is a vital undertaking that can lead to breakthroughs in treating, curing, and even preventing neurological and psychiatric diseases. By accelerating the development and application of innovative tools available to researchers today – such as the increasing resolution of imaging technologies and explosion of nanoscience (the study of very small matter such as atoms and molecules) – researchers hope to be able to produce a revolutionary dynamic picture of the brain whose level of detail has not yet been possible.

This brain image, which will show how individual cells and complex neural circuits interact in both time and space, will provide unprecedented understanding of how the brain enables the human body to record, process, utilize, store, and retrieve vast quantities of information, all at the speed of thought.

The NIH is working in close collaboration with other government agencies, including the Defense Advanced Research Agency and the National Science Foundation, as well as private partners, including the Allen Institute for Brain Science, the Howard Hughes Medical Institute, and the Kavli Foundation to achieve these profoundly ambitious goals.

The Banner Studies

The Banner Alzheimer's Institute, based in Phoenix, Arizona, is spearheading two drug trials involving genetic risk factors for Alzheimer's disease.

The first study, expected to begin in 2015, is called the **Alzheimer's Prevention Initiative** and will focus on late-onset Alzheimer's patients with two $APOE_4$ genes. With a grant awarded to them by the NIH, the Institute will test a drug (as yet to be determined) on 650 adults with two copies of the gene who have yet to show symptoms of cognitive decline.

To find the correct sampling of drug trial participants, Banner has created the Alzheimer's Prevention Registry to recruit volunteers who are willing to participate in medical studies. Volunteers in the Alzheimer's Prevention Registry will range from people with a family history of Alzheimer's, to those with a genetic predisposition for the disease, and those who are healthy. Within that pool of volunteers, researchers expect to find several hundred participants with two copies of $APOE_4$. The pharmaceutical industry, which has already invested hundreds of millions of dollars in failed attempts to create a preventative wonder drug, will take part in and help to fund the initiative in hopes of developing a treatment that successfully attacks the amyloid created by the $APOE_4$ gene.

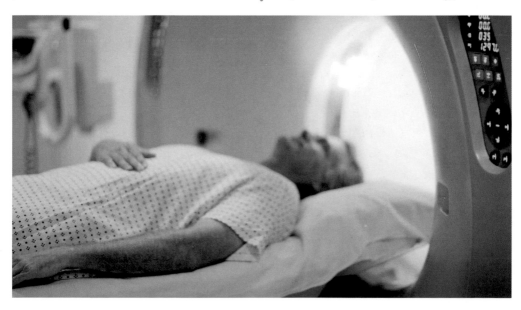

Banner aims to recruit up to 250,000 volunteers for the Alzheimer's Prevention Registry and plans to make the registry available to academic institutions and pharmaceutical companies who wish to conduct their own studies and prevention trials.

Banner's second drug trial is already underway in Colombia in collaboration with the biotechnology company Genentech, which manufactures the experimental drug *crenezumab* and is financing the largest portion of the trial. The study involves members of the largest extended family in the world to carry a gene mutation that guarantees early-onset Alzheimer's. 100 members of the Colombian family who carry a mutated version of the gene presenilin 1 will be given crenezumab, which removes plaque from the brain, while other members will take a placebo.

The Colombia trial is significant because it is testing a drug's effectiveness on subjects for which symptoms are guaranteed to emerge, while the Alzheimer's Prevention Initiative trial is significant for its focus on a much larger population at risk for the disease.

To Join the Alzheimer's Prevention Initiative: Visit www.endalznow.org and enter your email to become part of the Alzheimer's Prevention Registry. The registry is open to anyone aged 18 and older, of all races and ethnicities, with or without a family history of Alzheimer's disease.

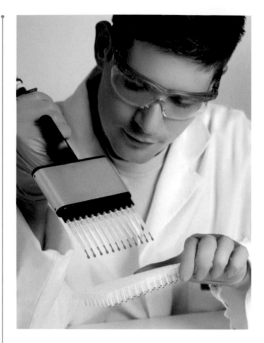

ADNI Initiative

The Alzheimer's Disease Neuroimaging Initiative (ADNI) was launched in 2004 by the NIH as the largest public-private partnership supporting Alzheimer's research. Its funding consortium includes pharmaceutical companies, science-related businesses, and non-profit organizations like the Alzheimer's Association. ADNI's original goal was to define biomarkers for use in clinical trials and to determine the best way to measure treatment effects of Alzheimer's. It is now in its third phase (ADNI 2), whose goal has been expanded to include the use of biomarkers to detect Alzheimer's at the pre-dementia stage, when treatments may be the most effective. ADNI 2 is taking place at 55 major academic medical centers and clinics in North America and the model is being adopted in other countries worldwide. ADNI 2 currently involves over 1000 study participants, including people without memory problems, those with mild cognitive impairment, and patients diagnosed with Alzheimer's.

ADNI maintains an unprecedented data access policy to encourage new investigation and to increase the pace of discovery of Alzheimer's treatments. All the data compiled by ADNI – including brain scans, blood and cerebrospinal fluid samples, and cognitive profiles of participants – is available to qualified scientists worldwide without embargo or delay, which has resulted in more than 500 scientific manuscripts thus far.

The "Big Data" project. At the 2013 Alzheimer's Association International Conference in Boston, Massachusetts, ADNI announced that massive amounts of data were available as a result of their first "Big Data" project for Alzheimer's disease, which was initiated as a collaboration between ADNI and the Brin Wojcicki Foundation. Whole genome sequencing was conducted on the largest cohort of individuals (more than 800 participants enrolled in ADNI) related to a single disease. The project has so far generated an estimated 200 terabytes of new genetic data.

Whole genome sequencing determines all six billion letters in an individual's DNA in one comprehensive analysis. The raw sequencing data is made available to the global scientific community so they may better understand how our genes cause and are affected by bodily changes associated with Alzheimer's disease.

Going Global. WW-ADNI (World Wide Alzheimer's Disease Neuroimaging Initiative) is the umbrella organization for neuroimaging initiatives being carried out through ADNI chapters around the world. In addition to the North American ADNI, global organizations include: E-ADNI (Europe), AIBL (Australia), Japan ADNI, Taiwan ADNI, Korea ADNI, China ADNI, and Argentina ADNI. Each WW-ADNI location collects participant data from MRI and PET scans as well as biomarker data and shares it across the international research community.

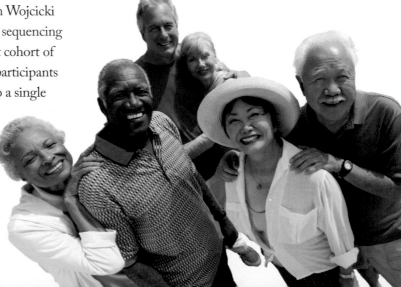

Global Alzheimer's Association Interactive Network (GAINN)

GAINN is a global data-sharing initiative similar in spirit and goals to ADNI's data access policy. It is built on an international database framework already in use by thousands of scientists and local computational facilities in North America and Europe. Via the Internet, the network makes data available free of charge for searching, downloading, and processing information from countless Alzheimer's studies. Researchers are able to link directly to their databases and add continually to their data sets, keeping GAINN data current and dynamic.

Participating in Clinical Trials and Epidemiological Studies

A clinical trial is a research study conducted on humans that rigorously tests the safety, side effects, and effectiveness of medication or behavioral treatments. The reason clinical trials and epidemiological studies are important is simple: New information leads to better treatment and prevention strategies.

Present-day medication only treats the symptoms, not the cause, of Alzheimer's disease, and no new drugs have been approved for Alzheimer's treatment since 2003, which makes clinical trials vital to the progress of diagnosing, treating, and stopping the disease. And databases like ADNI, GAINN and the Alzheimer's Prevention Initiative, which are discussed in the previous section, rely on volunteers to broaden their participant pools.

In randomized clinical trials, participants play different roles. Some participants are randomly selected to receive the intervention being tested, while others are given a placebo (a substance that has no pharmacological effect and acts as the control) and the differences in outcome that result from the trial are noted.

The value of any theory must be validated through multiple studies involving large groups of people, so the more people who participate, the more informative and convincing data becomes. Whether or not a person has Alzheimer's, volunteering to participate in clinical trials and other medical studies is a valuable contribution that will assist researchers and the medical community in helping Alzheimer's patients and their families.

ClinicalTrials.gov is a registry of federally and privately supported clinical trials. Users from around the world can search for clinical trials and find information about each trial's purpose, who may participate, locations, and other details. The website lists trials by country, indicates which of those trial are open for new participants, and provides contact information for volunteers to register.

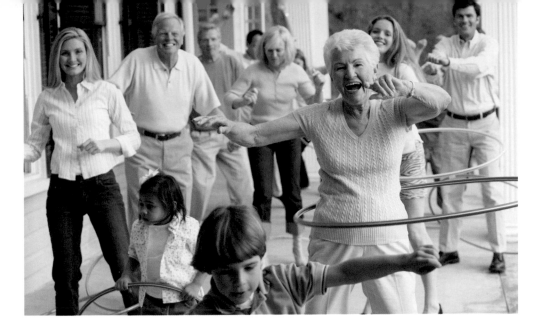

WHAT CAN WE DO IN THE MEANTIME?

Proactive Steps to Prevention

It is easy to become overwhelmed when confronted with so many facts and opinions about the current and future course of Alzheimer's disease. Until Alzheimer's can be prevented or cured, there will be certain unmodifiable factors – such as aging and genetics – whose effect is out of our hands.

But in the meantime, we can take control of our destiny by adopting a healthier lifestyle, among whose benefits may be the delay of Alzheimer's and MCI symptoms. We have the power to make the kinds of changes in our lives that will keep us healthy, engaged, and active, potentially staving off the disease indefinitely. Reducing a number of modifiable risk factors for Alzheimer's mitigates our risk for the disease. In Part II of this book, you will learn to empower yourself in the fight against Alzheimer's by implementing the following prevention strategies:

- Achieving and maintaining a healthy weight
- Addressing the symptoms of metabolic syndrome
- Reducing risk for type-2 diabetes
- Reducing risk for cardiovascular disease
- Engaging in physical activity (without risking head injury)
- Engaging in stimulating mental activity and positive social interaction.

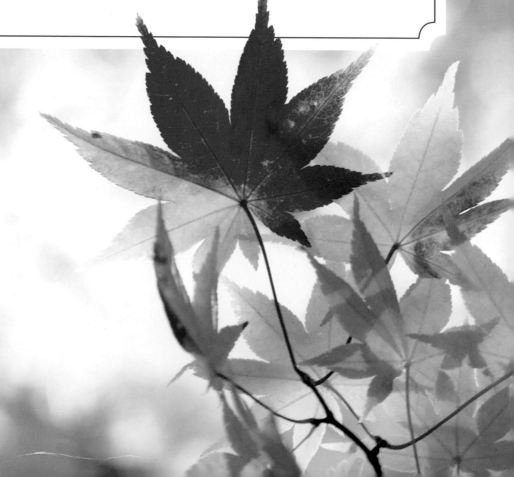

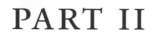

PART II
Preventing Alzheimer's:
How We Take Control

YOU CAN'T CHANGE your age, you can't change your gender, and you can't change your DNA – so what can you do to minimize your risk for Alzheimer's disease? The answer, which might seem simplistic, could be your best hope for prevention: Take care of your mind and body by eating right, exercising, and seeking out mental stimulation.

In Part I, you read that Alzheimer's disease shares a connection with common lifestyle conditions and diseases that can be prevented or controlled – namely, metabolic syndrome, heart disease, and type-2 diabetes. There are fairly simple changes you can implement and habits you can incorporate or remove from your daily life that go a long way in preventing these diseases and which scientists speculate in turn can prevent Alzheimer's.

You will also review the modifiable risk factors highlighted in the Dementia Risk Factor test – such as education/mental stimulation and physical activity – and learn strategies to incorporate such activities into your daily routine.

All individuals interested in improving their health – not just those at risk for developing chronic conditions like heart disease and diabetes – can benefit from the advice outlined in the following sections.

EATING AND WEIGHT LOSS

Maintaining a Healthy Weight

Reaching and maintaining a healthy weight is key to lowering your risk for chronic lifestyle-related diseases like heart disease and type-2 diabetes, as well as metabolic syndrome. As you learned in Part I of this guide, studies have shown that the symptoms of metabolic syndrome – obesity (particularly high abdominal fat), high blood pressure, elevated blood sugar, and high cholesterol – that lead to type-2 diabetes and heart disease can also be risk factors for Alzheimer's disease. Therefore, when you lose weight to prevent and control heart disease and type-2 diabetes, you are also doing your part to stave off Alzheimer's.

The key to losing weight and keeping it off is adopting a healthy lifestyle that includes regular exercise and a nutrition plan high in vitamins, minerals, and dietary fiber. Calorie count is secondary to the quality of the food you eat, so once you understand how your body operates and what it needs to operate efficiently, implementing simple lifestyle changes won't seem so daunting a task.

What is Metabolism?

"It's not my fault I'm overweight, I have a slow metabolism." Most of us have heard this rationalization or have been guilty of using it ourselves when our weight has crept up on us, seemingly without explanation. But what exactly is metabolism, and how does it affect your weight?

Metabolism is the term used to describe the chemical reactions involved in maintaining the living state of all cells in the human body, resulting in cell growth, production of energy, and elimination of waste. It is divided into two phases: catabolism and anabolism.

Catabolism, also called destructive metabolism, is the breakdown of complex substances into simpler ones, releasing energy in the process. Catabolism provides the energy your body needs for physical activity from the cellular level up to whole body movements. When you eat, catabolism breaks down nutrients and releases energy that is used in anabolism.

Anabolism, also called constructive metabolism, takes the energy produced in catabolism and synthesizes simple substances into more complex ones. Anabolic reactions use chemicals and molecules to grow new cells that build things like bones and muscles and maintain all the tissues in your body.

In other words, the food you eat provides the calories (energy) that stimulate catabolic and anabolic function. Food contains essential nutrients (those which the body cannot produce on its own) necessary for the efficient function of the body.

- **Carbohydrates**: Carbohydrates come in three forms. Two forms, starches and sugars, are converted to glucose during metabolism. Body tissue depends on glucose for all activities. Fiber, a third carbohydrate, passes through your system undigested and helps your body eliminate waste.
- **Proteins**: Proteins are the body's main tissue builders and come from meat, eggs, dairy products, soybeans, vegetables, and grains.
- **Fat**: The vital functions of fat include helping to form cells, cushioning and insulating organs, helping to absorb fat-soluble vitamins, and providing reserve stores of energy.
- **Vitamins and Minerals**: Although they don't provide calories on their own, vitamins and minerals are nutrients that the body needs to grow and develop properly. Vitamins come from organic substances (plants or animals), and minerals are inorganic elements found in the soil and water that are absorbed by plants. Eating a balanced diet of carbohydrates,

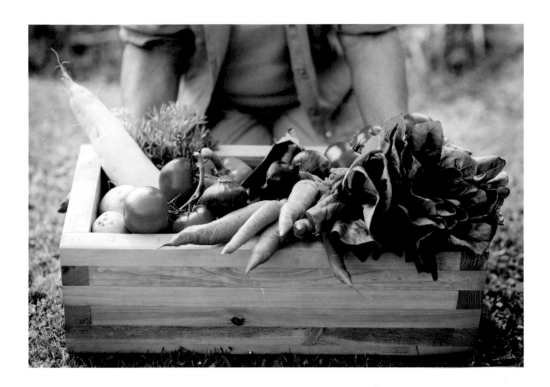

proteins, and fats provides all the daily vitamins a person needs, without having to take supplements.

Body weight is determined by the amount of carbohydrates, proteins, and fats you eat on a daily basis, subtracting anabolism (energy out) from catabolism (energy in). When the resulting quantity is negative (more calories out than in) you lose weight. When the resulting quantity is positive (more calories in than out) you gain weight. To maintain weight, the calories going in must equal the energy going out to achieve energy balance. You need to eat to obtain energy and maintain a healthy body, but if you eat more food than you need, producing more energy than you use up, you gain weight.

The body stores excess energy as fat. Fat tissue is relatively inactive compared to muscle or organ tissue and other systems in your body. And fat cells, because of their relative inactivity, do not require much energy to maintain themselves. Thus, active people with more muscle need more calories than inactive people with more fat because muscles require more energy to grow. To burn fat and increase lean muscle mass you need to exercise.

As you age, several factors lower your calorie requirements. Your muscle-to-fat ratio changes as muscle mass drops due to one or more of the following:

- **Hormones:** Men produce less testosterone and women less estrogen, which are hormones involved in anabolic processes that consume energy.
- **Menopause:** As women transition into menopause and post-menopause, weight gain is partially related to a drop in anabolic hormone production.
- **Physical Activity:** In general, our level of physical activity drops as we age. This is partially due to leisurely lifestyle activities, as well as the type of jobs people tend to have later in their career. Either due to promotions or because of protocol, work situations tend to become more sedentary as we age.
- **Lower Basal Metabolic Rate:** Basal metabolic rate (BMR) is the rate that energy is expended while the body is at rest. As we age, our BMR decreases and we tend to lose lean body mass, making it more difficult to burn calories. If we continue to eat the same amount of calories per day as our BMR decreases, we gain weight.

Watching what you eat each day – without being severely restrictive – and staying physically active are key to maintaining a healthy body weight as you age. A healthy, well-balanced diet that assists the metabolic process should include whole grains, fruits and vegetables, lean proteins, and calcium, as well as fats and sugars from good sources.

You don't need to be a vigilant calorie counter to be healthy. What you need to understand is that the more you move and the better you eat, the closer you will be to your ideal weight, which will result in long-term health benefits. Nutrition-wise, what's most important is that you eat a well-balanced diet of quality food.

If you feel yourself putting on excess pounds, you can make adjustments like reducing the portion size of your food, eating more vegetables and less meat or moving more each day to burn off the excess calories.

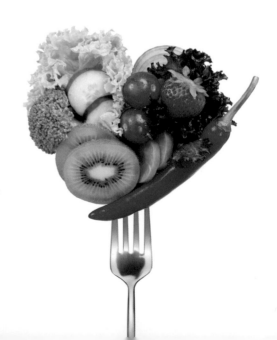

DIET MISTAKES THAT SABOTAGE METABOLISM

✔ **Eating Refined Carbohydrates:** The kind of starch and fiber you eat matters. Refined carbohydrates like white flour, white sugar, and white rice convert easily to fat. Switching to whole grains and eating plenty of fruits, vegetables, and legumes, which also contain dietary fiber, can increase the rate at which your body burns fat and eliminates waste.

✔ **Not Enough Protein:** Protein should be a component of every meal you eat. Your body needs protein to maintain lean muscle mass. If you are skimping on proteins because you are trying to stay away from animal fat, seek out vegetarian options like nuts, seeds, and beans.

✔ **Your Diet Lacks Iron:** Iron helps your blood pump oxygen to your muscles, which use it to burn fat. Shellfish, lean meat, beans, and spinach are excellent sources of iron. Older adults and people who follow a vegan diet are more susceptible to iron deficiency, but there could be other serious underlying causes. Before turning to an iron supplement or overcompensating with iron-rich foods, have your blood count and iron level checked. If it is low, your doctor can identify the reason for the deficiency and recommend an appropriate course of action, which might include eating iron-rich foods or a daily vitamin supplement. ***Take Note**: Iron supplements are not instant metabolism boosters, so don't run to the vitamin shop to stock up.

✔ **Drinking to Excess:** Reducing your alcohol intake is an easy way to shed a few pounds. When you drink, instead of reaching to your fat stores for energy, your body uses the alcohol as fuel – the more alcohol you drink, the less fat you burn. Moreover, alcoholic beverages are high in calories, so limit your alcohol intake to keep your metabolism on track and your weight down.

✔ **Not Eating Enough:** Yes, you can eat too little. When you eat less per day than your body requires for basic function, your metabolic rate goes into protection mode and actually slows down in order to store more energy as fat to compensate for the calorie deficiency. Make sure that you don't go hungry during the day, and snack on fruit, yogurt, or nuts between meals to sustain your metabolic rate.

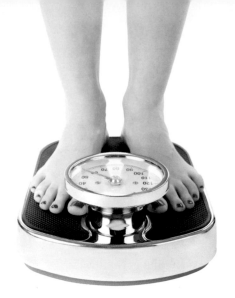

Weight Loss and Nutrition Myths

FAD DIETS WORK

The short answer is no. Fad diets often promise extreme and swift results but they rarely take healthful eating habits and long term health and weight maintenance goals into account. At first, weight loss may be rapid, but these diets are usually unrealistic and difficult to follow, so people abandon them, putting the weight back on and then some. In certain cases, the weight loss regimen is so extreme that people lose too much weight at once, which can result in gallstones and even serious heart problems. If good health is the number one goal of your weight loss regimen, then sensible lifestyle changes will carry you through.

MYTH 2 SOME PEOPLE CAN EAT WHATEVER THEY WANT AND NOT GAIN WEIGHT

It might seem that way when you see a thin person eating portion sizes much larger than your own or calorie-laden foods that you do your best to avoid – but it isn't so. The metabolic equation of calories in minus energy out applies to everyone. No one can stay thin eating all the cheeseburgers and pizzas they want without burning all the calories that come with them. Chances are, people who seem like they can eat anything they want exercise regularly and have a good ratio of lean muscle mass to fat, as well as a high basal metabolism – the rate at which the body burns calories while at rest. Basal metabolic rate varies among individuals, and those with higher BMRs

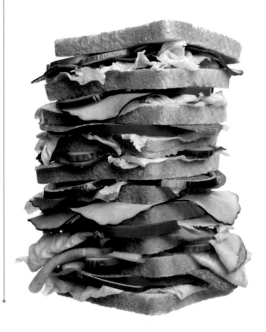

require more calories per day for their bodies to perform basic life functions. Moreover, everyone, no matter their BMR, needs to consume healthful foods in order to reduce their risk for lifestyle diseases, so the quality of your calorie intake is paramount – even thin people should keep the cheeseburgers and pizzas to a minimum.

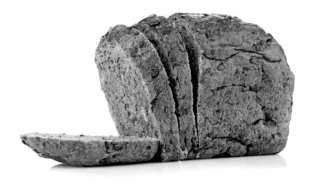

MYTH 3 — CARBOHYDRATES ARE FATTENING SO I SHOULD AVOID THEM

Carbohydrates are your body's main energy source, so it is not advisable to cut them out of your diet. Eating too few carbohydrates can lead to malnutrition and an excessive intake of fats to compensate for the loss in calories. The important thing to keep in mind is the quality of the carbohydrates you eat. There are two main types of carbohydrates – simple carbohydrates, categorized as sugars, and complex carbohydrates, categorized as starches and fibers. Simple carbs consist of just one or two sugar molecules, while complex carbs consist of more complicated strings of sugar molecules. Foods high in complex carbohydrates are good sources of dietary fiber, vitamins, and minerals and take longer to break down, while simple carb options – like cakes, candies, cookies, and soft drinks – are digested quickly, providing many calories but few nutrients. Eating whole fruits and vegetables, legumes, nuts and seeds, as well as unrefined or "whole" grains like brown rice and whole-wheat bread, is the way to go.

Foods high in complex carbohydrates are good sources of dietary fiber, vitamins, and minerals and take longer to break down.

MYTH 4 — 'LOW FAT' OR 'FAT FREE' MEANS I CAN EAT AS MUCH AS I WANT

Foods are often packaged and sold as low or non-fat as a way to lure health-conscious customers into purchasing them. But just because a food is low-fat or fat-free doesn't mean it is calorie-free or even nutritious. As with any food, serving size and ingredients matter. In fact, one serving of the fat-free version of a food might have even more calories than one serving of its original, full-fat counterpart. Low-fat or fat-free foods often require the addition of simple carbs to compensate for the taste and texture of the fat that has been removed. Always remember to read labels, not only for calorie count and serving size, but also for ingredients. Packaged foods labeled "healthy" or "fat-free" usually contain the kinds of ingredients you should avoid.

MYTH 5 — SKIPPING MEALS HELPS ME LOSE WEIGHT

Just the opposite. Studies actually show a link between skipping meals, particularly breakfast, and obesity. On average, people who skip breakfast tend to be heavier than those who eat breakfast. Regularly skipping meals can slow down your metabolism because the longer you wait between meals, the longer your body is in sleep mode, burning fewer calories. Also, people who skip a meal tend to overcompensate at the next one, senselessly eating too much of whatever is put in front of them and ingesting too many calories in the process.

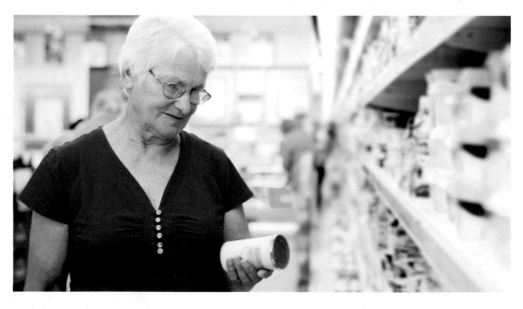

Weight Loss Principles – Learn to eat differently for life

✔ Weight loss is recommended for overweight and obese people in order to prevent or control lifestyle disease and conditions such as high blood pressure, high cholesterol, type-2 diabetes, heart disease, and metabolic syndrome.

✔ Decreasing abdominal fat in particular is essential to staving off many lifestyle diseases.

✔ Implement reasonable lifestyle changes to your diet and exercise routines to stay healthy – obsessive calorie counting and deprivation can and will undermine healthy weight goals.

✔ To lose weight, you must burn more calories than you consume in a day.

✔ To maintain a healthy weight, you must achieve energy balance, where the number of calories going in equals the energy going out on average over time.

✔ Reducing dietary fat intake alone, without reducing overall calorie intake, is not sufficient for weight loss.

✔ Physical activity, to the extent possible, should be a part of any weight loss and weight maintenance program.

✔ Lean muscle burns more calories than fat. Add strength training to your exercise plan to increase your lean muscle mass and burn calories even when you are at rest.

✔ Small changes to your eating habits can make a big difference. Gradually introduce new, healthful foods into your diet while eliminating less healthy options, and before long you will look and feel better.

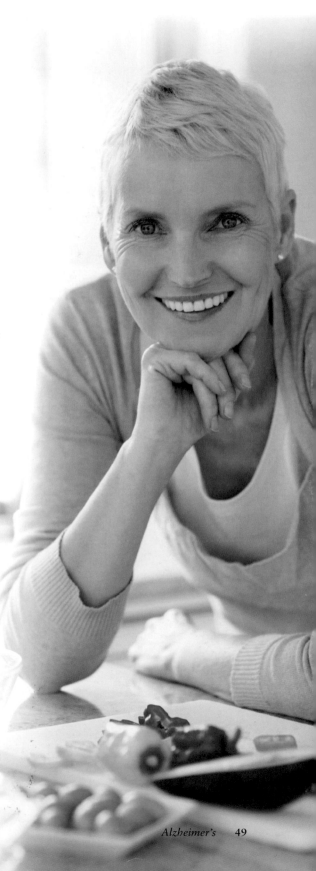

HEALTHY EATING OPTIONS TO PREVENT AND CONTROL TYPE-2 DIABETES, HIGH BLOOD PRESSURE, AND HEART DISEASE

A Note About Dietary Supplements

The recommendations in this guide are for food sources of nutrients only. Although essential nutrients can be obtained through supplementary means, the effectiveness of vitamin and mineral supplements has met much scrutiny lately. Moreover, taking supplements can adversely interact with medical conditions and medications, so it's best to consult your physician before introducing them to your nutrition plan.

If you do take supplements, they should not be considered a substitute for food, which should be your main source of nutrients and dietary fiber.

Eating to Prevent and Control Type-2 Diabetes

* Please note: If you have already been diagnosed with type-2 diabetes, do not abandon any prescriptions or advice from your doctor in favor of switching to a glycemic index-based diet or any other diet – it is important that you follow your doctor's instructions for insulin and drug interventions. Consulting with your doctor and/or registered dietitian will help you make informed choices when changing your diet and exercise habits so that you do not to compromise your medical treatment or your health.

The majority of people who are diagnosed with type-2 diabetes are

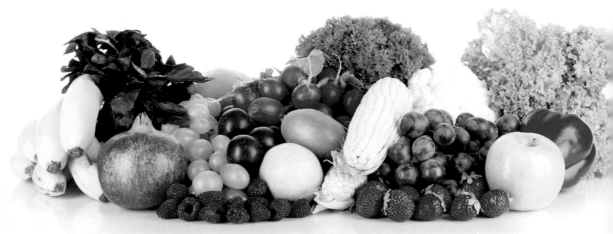

overweight. The more overweight you are, the higher at risk you are. Excessive weight around your midsection in particular is a major risk factor for type-2 diabetes. Moreover, people at risk for type-2 diabetes are also much more likely to develop cardiovascular complications such as coronary artery disease, high blood pressure, and stroke.

Diet and exercise are key to reducing the belly fat that leads to type-2 diabetes. Following a Mediterranean-style diet, which is described further along in this chapter, and doing aerobic exercise at least three times per week will help you lose weight, particularly around your midsection. Another diet element to consider is the glycemic load of the food you eat.

What are Glycemic Index and Glycemic Load?

Glucose is the sugar that provides the primary means of energy for all the body's cells. The main source of glucose is carbohydrates. During digestion, your pancreas produces insulin, a digestive hormone that helps your body's cells absorb glucose from the blood. The insulin is released when glucose is present in the blood – without insulin, glucose cannot enter your cells, and

without glucose, your cells would not be able to function.

In type-2 diabetes, high levels of glucose in the blood are not being absorbed, either because the body cannot produce enough insulin or because it is insulin resistant, meaning that the insulin is no longer effective at reducing blood glucose. When you apply glycemic index/glycemic load principles to your diet, you can help to control the amount of excess glucose in your blood.

There are two kinds of carbohydrates – simple and complex. Simple carbohydrates are found in refined sugars, refined grains, and fruits. Simple carbs digest quickly, causing spikes in blood glucose levels. On food labels

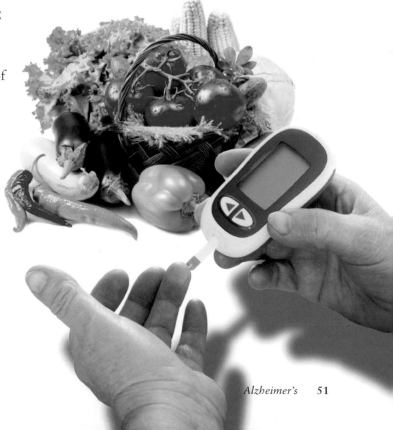

they might be listed as glucose, sucrose, lactose, or fructose. Examples of simple carbohydrates are: table sugar, corn syrup, white flour, jellies, jams, milk, ice cream, soda, white rice, processed snack foods, and packaged cereals.

Complex carbohydrates are called starches and are composed of simple carbohydrates that are chemically bonded together. Due to their complexity, they take longer to digest, thus helping to regulate blood glucose levels. Complex carbohydrates are typically found in vegetables, legumes, and whole grains. Examples of complex carbohydrates are: spinach, lentils, broccoli, whole grain bread, whole wheat pasta, potatoes, yams, and wild rice.

Fiber is characterized as a type of complex carbohydrate, but it does not act like other carbs. Fiber is the indigestible part of plant foods like fruits, vegetables, grains, nuts, and legumes. Eating fiber promotes regular digestion and elimination of waste, and can lower cholesterol levels. Sources of dietary fiber include: beans and legumes like black beans, kidney beans, chick peas, lentils; fruits and vegetables with edible skin and edible seeds like apples, grapes, and berries; whole grain cereals and breads; whole grain pasta; and all varieties of nuts.

You need to eat carbohydrates to survive, but you should be aware of the quality of carbohydrates you consume in order to reduce your belly fat and excess glucose in your blood stream, thus reducing your risk for type-2 diabetes. Glycemic index principles do not involve extreme low-carb or low-fat diet methods or calorie counting. Instead, they indicate how the type of carbohydrate you eat has an effect on blood glucose. As a general rule, complex carbohydrates are preferable to simple carbohydrates.

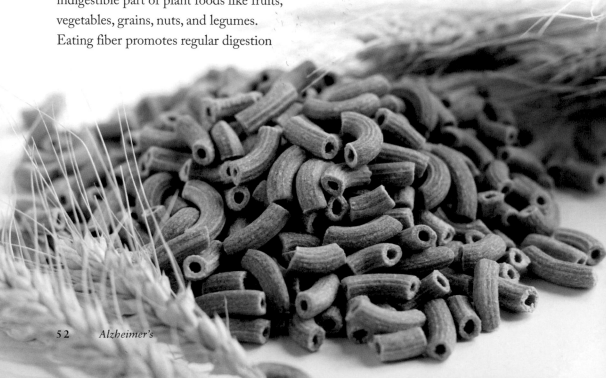

The glycemic index is a numerical scale that measures the quality of carbohydrates in foods and shows how fast the carbs in a particular food can raise blood sugar (glucose.) The index ranks foods and beverages on a scale from 0 to 100. Only foods and beverages that contain carbs are ranked – meats and fats don't have a GI ranking because on their own, they do not contain carbohydrates. Low-ranked foods have a score of 55 or under. Foods in the middle of the scale rank 56-69. Foods with a GI score of 70 or higher rank the highest on the scale.

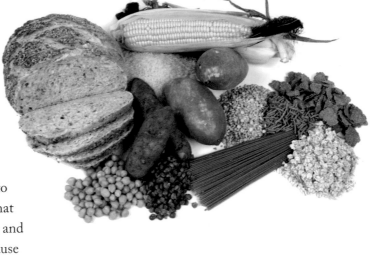

Low GI foods are considered the most desirable because they take longer to digest, control appetite and delay hunger pangs, which helps with weight management. Your body digests high GI foods most rapidly, causing your blood glucose levels to spike. Blood glucose spikes are often followed by huge dips. These fluctuations in your blood sugar can lead to hormonal imbalance, mood swings, elevated blood pressure, fatigue, trembling, and binge eating.

The concept of glycemic load fine-tunes glucose management because it uses portion size in combination with glycemic index to determine the effect of a particular food on your blood glucose level. In other words, glycemic load measures how high a serving of food raises your blood sugar, so the amount of food you eat matters just as much as its GI. Meal planning using glycemic index as a guide involves eating food in portion sizes and combinations that result a low or medium glycemic load score. Or, when eating a high GI food, combining it with a low GI food to counteract its effect.

Sticking to low or medium-range glycemic load foods is recommended, but according to glycemic load charts, eating a small amount of a high GI food that contains essential nutrients is acceptable, whereas eating large amounts of a low GI food can raise its glycemic load to an unacceptable level.

Many foods are naturally low on the glycemic index, so if you already eat a sensible diet full of fresh fruits and vegetables, avoiding highly processed foods and refined grains, chances are that you are in control of your blood glucose. But if you need a little extra guidance, you can find free information on the glycemic index and free glycemic load charts by conducting an Internet search. There are also several glycemic index guides in print that you can find at your local library or purchase from a local or online book retailer.

Things to Consider When Using the Glycemic Index

✔ Glycemic index and glycemic load are dietary tools for controlling blood glucose. They are not a diet plan.

✔ Glycemic index and glycemic load charts help you choose the right carbs, they do not advocate a low or no-carb lifestyle.

✔ You control glucose intake by portion size not calorie count.

✔ A food high on the glycemic index might have a relatively low glycemic load score when portion size is taken into account.

✔ The GI of a food is different when eaten alone than when it is combined with other foods.

✔ Many nutritious foods have a higher GI than some with little nutritional value, so it is important to use common sense when making food choices. You can pair healthful high GI foods with healthful low GI foods to balance your meal.

✔ The more ripe a fruit or vegetable is, the higher its GI.

✔ The more processed a food is, the higher its GI – mashed potatoes have a higher GI than a whole baked potato and juice has a higher GI than whole fruit, for example.

✔ Cooking time affects GI. For instance, al dente pasta has a lower GI than pasta that is cooked soft.

Examples of Food Swaps for Lowering Glycemic Index

INSTEAD OF...	EAT...
White rice	Brown or wild rice
Semolina pasta	Whole wheat pasta
Instant oatmeal	Steel cut oats
Cornflakes	Bran flakes
Mashed potatoes	Baked yams
Apple Sauce	Whole apple
Soda	Tomato juice
Alcohol	Water

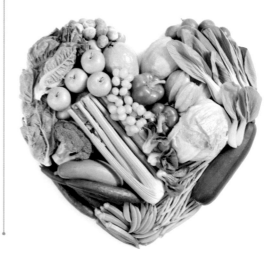

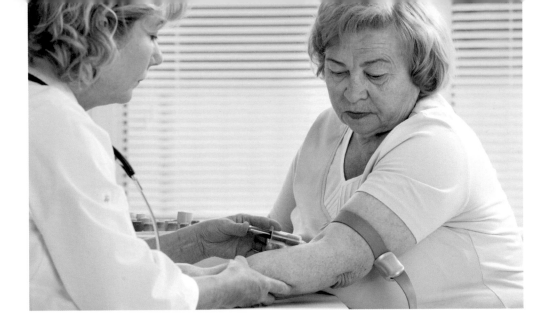

What is High Cholesterol?

Every cell in the human body contains cholesterol in its outer layer. Cholesterol is vital for normal body function – it builds and maintains cell membranes, insulates nerve fibers, produces hormones, aids in the production of bile, converts sunlight to vitamin D, and metabolizes fat-soluble vitamins, including A, D, E, and K. So if cholesterol does so much good, what does it mean to have a cholesterol problem?

Cholesterol is transported through the blood by molecules called lipoproteins – compounds that contain both lipids (fats) and proteins. There are three main kinds of lipoproteins: low density lipoprotein (LDL), high density lipoprotein (HDL), and triglycerides. LDL is often referred to as "bad" cholesterol because if there is too much LDL for cells to use, it builds up as plaque in the arteries and increases risk for heart disease. Conversely, HDL is often referred to as "good" cholesterol because it helps to fight against heart disease by removing LDL cholesterol from where it does not belong and transporting it to the liver where it is broken down.

Triglycerides work together with cholesterol to form plasma lipids (blood fat.) Triglycerides originate from fats in food or are formed within the body using food sources such as carbohydrates. Calories that are not immediately used by body tissue are converted into triglycerides and stored in fat cells for later use when the body needs energy. Regularly eating more calories than you burn can result in high triglycerides, and the types of food you eat determine your cholesterol level. In other words, diet and exercise are key to controlling LDL and triglyceride levels.

Problems associated with high LDL include: atherosclerosis (narrowing of the arteries); coronary artery disease; angina (chest pain); heart attack, and stroke. If both LDL and triglyceride levels are too high, the risk of developing coronary artery disease rises significantly.

Simple blood tests can measure your cholesterol and triglycerides, and the good news is that a change in lifestyle habits is often all you need to bring them back down to desirable levels.

Explaining Omega-3 Fatty Acids

Essential nutrients are nutrients that the body cannot make on its own and must be obtained from a dietary source or supplement. Omega-3 fatty acids are essential nutrients that reduce inflammation and may lower risk of chronic diseases such as heart disease and diabetes. Omega-3s are highly concentrated in the brain and are important for cognitive and behavioral function. Symptoms of omega-3 deficiency include fatigue, poor memory, dry skin, heart problems, mood swings or depression, and poor circulation.

Food sources for omega-3s include fish, plant, and nut oils. Eicosapentaenoic (EPA) and dcocahexaenoic (DHA) acids – two essential omega 3s – are found in cold water fish such as salmon, mackerel, halibut, sardines, tuna, and herring. Alpha-linolenic acid (ALA), another type of omega-3, is found in flaxseeds, flaxseed oil, canola oil, pumpkin seeds, pumpkin seed oil, walnuts, and walnut oil.

Like omega-3s, omega-6 fatty acids are essential nutrients, but most omega-6 fatty acids tend to promote inflammation rather than reduce it. We often consume too many omega-6s and not enough omega-3s because of the amount of processed foods we eat, so it is important to consume the proper ratio of omega-3 foods to omega-6 foods. A Mediterranean-style diet is an ideal example of a food plan that addresses this concern.

Omega-3 fatty acids have been shown to be beneficial to the following conditions.

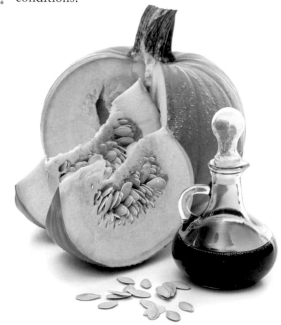

✔ **Heart disease:** The role of omega-3 fatty acids in cardiovascular disease are well established. Clinical evidence suggests that EPA and DHA help reduce risk factors for heart disease, including high cholesterol and high blood pressure. Omega-3s obtained from fish lower triglyceride levels, and lower the risk of heart attack, stroke, and abnormal heart rhythm in people who have already had a heart attack. They also help to prevent and treat atherosclerosis. Eating at least two servings of fish per week can reduce the risk of stroke by 50%.

✔ **High cholesterol:** High levels of HDL (good cholesterol) help promote heart health. People who get high amounts of omega-3 fatty acids from fish tend to have increased HDL and decreased triglycerides. Also, walnuts, which are high in ALA, have been reported to lower total cholesterol and triglycerides in people with high cholesterol levels.

✔ **High blood pressure:** Studies suggest that diets rich in omega-3s lower blood pressure in people with hypertension.

✔ **Diabetes:** People with diabetes often have high triglycerides and low HDL levels. Eating omega-3-rich fish can help regulate cholesterol levels and lower apoproteins – markers of diabetes; however, ALA may not have the same effect as EPA and DHA in diabetes patients because some people with diabetes cannot convert ALA to the EPA or DHA forms of omega-3 that the body can use.

✔ **Cognitive Decline:** Studies show that a diet low in omega-3 fatty acids results in an increased risk for age-related cognitive decline and dementia, including Alzheimer's disease. Scientists believe that DHA in particular is a protective factor for Alzheimer's.

DHA and Alzheimer's

DHA is one of the major building blocks of the brain in all stages of life. It is crucial for neurological and visual development in infants and plays a role in the ongoing structure and function of the adult brain. In recent studies, DHA has been shown to reduce the risk of Alzheimer's disease in people who eat at least one serving of fish per week. People with Alzheimer's have dramatically lower levels of DHA in the neurons of the hippocampus – one of the first parts of the brain to be affected by the disease.

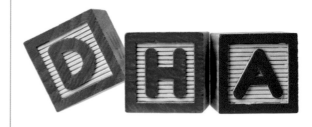

Mediterranean Diet for Heart Health, Weight Loss, and Weight Maintenance

A Mediterranean-style eating plan is easy to follow because it doesn't ban entire food groups, and the variety of foods available is both enjoyable and satisfying to eat. It is based on the eating habits of the European countries that border the Mediterranean Sea.

There is not one specific Mediterranean diet – the Italians eat differently from the Spanish, who eat differently from the Greeks, and so on. What matters are certain commonalities that these populations share – an emphasis on fruits, vegetables, fish, poultry, and legumes; a use of flavorful herbs and spices; a preference for olive oil over butter and whole grains over refined carbohydrates; and moderate red wine consumption. Red meat, saturated fats and sweets are eaten sparingly, and food is baked, broiled, grilled, roasted or boiled, but rarely fried.

While many sensible diet plans advocate eating lots of fruits, vegetables, and whole grains, following a Mediterranean-style diet in particular is associated with a reduced risk of death from heart disease and cancer, as well as with reduced levels of inflammation and instance of Alzheimer's disease. Because a Mediterranean-style diet features omega-3-rich foods, it can reduce LDL (bad cholesterol,) and because it emphasizes whole grains, it is a good option for people trying to regulate blood glucose and lose belly fat.

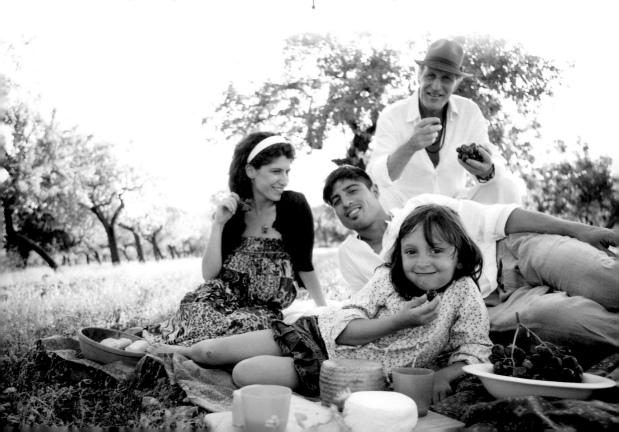

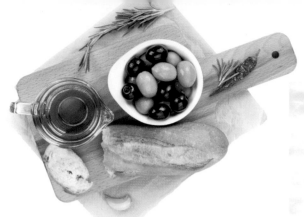

Basic Mediterranean Diet Guidelines

- Eat vegetables at every meal – aim for 3-8 servings a day.
- Eat fruits, whole grains, beans, legumes, nuts, and herbs and spices every day.
- Eat omega-3-rich fish and seafood often, at least twice a week.
- Eat moderate portions of poultry, eggs, cheese, and yogurt.
- Eat fatty red meat sparingly, no more than a few times a month.
- Have fruit for dessert and save the sweets for special occasions.
- Cook with olive oil as often as possible, but do not fry your food.
- Don't butter your bread. Mediterranean cultures dip their bread in olive oil.
- Drink a glass (or two, on occasion) of red wine a day.
- Snack on nuts, seeds, or low-fat dairy products rather than processed snack foods.
- Slow down – people in Mediterranean cultures take time to savor their food so that they eat until they are satisfied rather than stuffed.

THE BENEFITS OF RED WINE

- ✔ It may lower LDL or "bad" cholesterol.
- ✔ It may help maintain heart health.
- ✔ Is a source of resveratrol – an antioxidant that has been shown to help regulate blood sugar and hamper the formation of beta-amyloid.

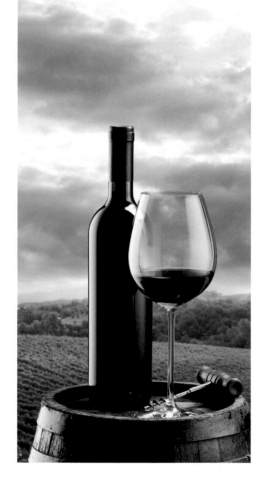

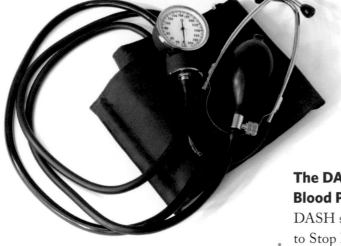

The DASH Diet to Lower Blood Pressure

DASH stands for Dietary Approaches to Stop Hypertension (high blood pressure.) In addition to its main emphasis of lowering high blood pressure, much like the Mediterranean diet, the DASH diet is a lifestyle approach to food that advocates healthy eating to prevent and control lifestyle diseases like heart disease, stroke, high cholesterol, and diabetes.

Unlike the Mediterranean diet, the full DASH plan is based on a calorie system that is determined by your age and activity level. The more you move, the more food you can eat to maintain your weight – a sedentary 60-year-old female requires fewer total calories than a moderately active 40-year-old female, for example. And the calorie requirements are met by following a diet plan that calls for a specific number of servings from each food group per day. If you want to learn more about the full DASH eating plan, more information is available from the National Heart, Lung, and Blood Institute (USA) website at www.nhlbi.nih.gov.

What is High Blood Pressure?

Blood pressure is the force at which your heart pumps blood through your arteries. It is measured in two numbers. The top number measures *systolic* pressure, which is the force created when the heart beats. The bottom number represents the force created when the heart relaxes between beats, called *diastolic* pressure.

Normal blood pressure is less than 120 systolic and 80 diastolic, written as 120/80. High blood pressure, also called hypertension, occurs when blood pressure measurements regularly exceed 140/90.

High blood pressure overtaxes your heart by making it pump harder to force your blood to circulate. If it remains uncontrolled, high blood pressure can lead to heart and kidney disease, stroke, and even blindness. High blood pressure is one of the symptoms of metabolic syndrome and is also one of the Alzheimer's risk factors highlighted in the Dementia Risk Factor test, which is discussed in Part I of this book.

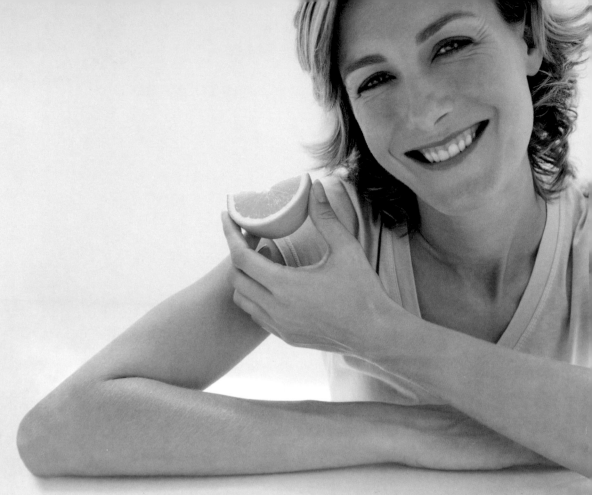

General Guidelines for Transitioning to the DASH Lifestyle

- Limit lean meats to two 3-ounce (85g) portions per day. One 3-ounce portion of meat is about equal in size to a deck of cards.
- Gradually add a serving of vegetables to each meal.
- Add fruit to one meal and eat fruit as a snack.
- Eat at least two vegetarian-style meals per week.
- Eat whole grain pasta and brown rice.
- Cook with bagged dry beans. Canned beans are preserved with sodium.

- When not cooking with fresh vegetables, bagged frozen vegetables are preferable to canned.
- Eat unsalted nuts.
- Season your food with something other than salt at the table. Lemon juice and vinegar make good salt substitutes, as do flavorful herbs and spices, but avoid seasoning mixes that contain salt.
- Read food labels – foods with 20% or more suggested daily value of sodium are considered high.

HIGH-SODIUM FOODS TO AVOID

✔ Heat-and-serve meals (frozen dinners)

✔ Canned meats

✔ Canned soups

✔ Canned vegetables and beans

✔ Bottled vegetable juices

✔ Bottled salad dressing

✔ Cured meats like hot dogs, bacon, salami, and luncheon meat

✔ Condiments like ketchup and steak sauce

✔ Jarred spaghetti sauce

✔ Bagged snack foods like potato chips, corn chips and pretzels

✔ Soy sauce

✔ Powdered broths and gravies

✔ Bouillon cubes

✔ Ramen noodle flavor packets

✔ Yeast extract spreads like Marmite and Vegemite

✔ Fast food items

✔ Soda

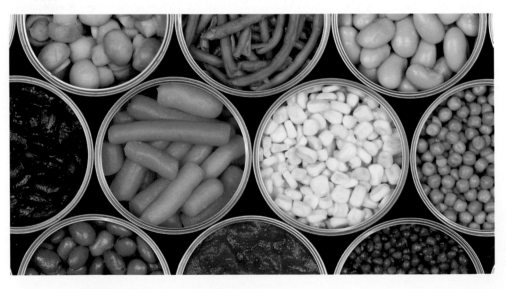

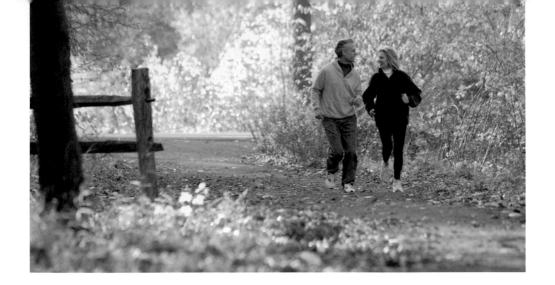

What is Inflammation?

As explained in Part I, inflammation is your immune system's response to external attack, such as a cut or a virus. Acute inflammation disappears when conditions are treated; however, chronic inflammation can harm your body because it doesn't shut off easily. With chronic inflammation, immune cells constantly attack healthy tissue, resulting in an array of diseases and conditions such as cancer, diabetes, heart disease, stroke, and even Alzheimer's disease.

Risk factors for chronic inflammation include:

- **Being overweight:** Carrying too much weight, particularly around the midsection, is a sign that your body is producing too many pro-inflammatory chemicals – substances in your body that promote inflammation, making a disease worse and accelerating the aging process. Fat cells that accumulate around the organs in your abdominal cavity are reacting to the stress hormone cortisol, which causes them to produce more chemicals that increase inflammation.

- **Metabolic Syndrome:** A combination of high blood pressure, high glucose levels, and high triglycerides are signs that your body is inflamed and at risk for diabetes and heart disease.

- **Inactivity:** A sedentary lifestyle promotes inflammation. Working out 60 minutes a day can protect against metabolic syndrome.

- **Stress:** Stress can cause belly fat to accumulate.

- **Lack of Sleep:** The body requires 7-8 hours of sleep per night to reduce stress.

- **Poor Dental Hygiene:** Scientists have found that the bacteria that causes inflammation in gums is the same bacteria that is a source of inflammation and thickening of the arteries.

Eating to Control Chronic Inflammation

The anti-inflammatory diet asserts that what you eat can determine how much inflammation you produce – certain foods promote inflammation, while others help to fight it. A full anti-inflammation eating plan has been created by Dr. Andrew Weil, a medical doctor and naturopath based in the United States who has written extensively on holistic health. Dr. Weil established the field of integrative medicine, which combines the principles of conventional and alternative medicine to achieve optimum health. You can find Dr. Weil's anti-inflammatory eating plan outlined on his website at **www.drweil.com**.

You can incorporate the following anti-inflammation guidelines as part of your overall healthy eating plan.

OPT FOR...

- ✔ Omega-3-rich foods like salmon and tuna, walnuts and other nuts, flaxseeds and flaxseed oil, and canola oil
- ✔ Colorful produce like red onions, tomatoes, broccoli, red grapes, berries, and oranges
- ✔ Beans and legumes
- ✔ Cooked mushrooms
- ✔ Lean, skinless white meat
- ✔ Dark chocolate – at least 70% cacao
- ✔ Unsweetened dried fruit
- ✔ Red wine
- ✔ Green tea
- ✔ Ginger
- ✔ Turmeric
- ✔ Rosemary
- ✔ Garlic

TRY TO AVOID...

- ✖ Omega-6 fats like corn, safflower, and vegetable oils; mayonnaise, and bottled salad dressing
- ✖ Trans fats – read nutrition labels to make sure products do not contain any percentage of trans fat
- ✖ Rancid fats – heating oils to the point when the smoke causes fats to oxidize, making them inflammation boosters; old peanut butter and chocolate that have been stashed in the pantry for years have also oxidized and should be avoided
- ✖ White starches like bleached flour, white rice, and instant mashed potatoes cause spikes in blood sugar levels that result in inflammation
- ✖ Excess alcohol – having more than two drinks a day can cause changes in the intestinal lining, allowing bacteria to pass into the blood stream, triggering inflammation

GOOD FOOD TIPS

Foods That Boost Brain Power

- **Fatty Fish**: Fish like salmon, albacore tuna, mackerel, herring, and sardines are loaded with nutrient-rich omega-3 fatty acids that help reduce inflammation and cholesterol and help lower the risk for heart disease. DHA is a fatty acid found in cold water fish. It is often used as a supplement to treat coronary artery disease, type-2 diabetes, and dementia. It plays a key role in the development of nerve tissue, decreases blood thickness, and lowers triglycerides. Some research suggests that getting more DHA from the diet might help prevent Alzheimer's.

- **Berries:** Berries are an antioxidant super-fruit. Try incorporating your favorite berries – blueberries, strawberries, cranberries and acai berries are highest in antioxidants – into your morning cereal or oatmeal and adding them to plain yogurt for a healthy snack at least once a day.

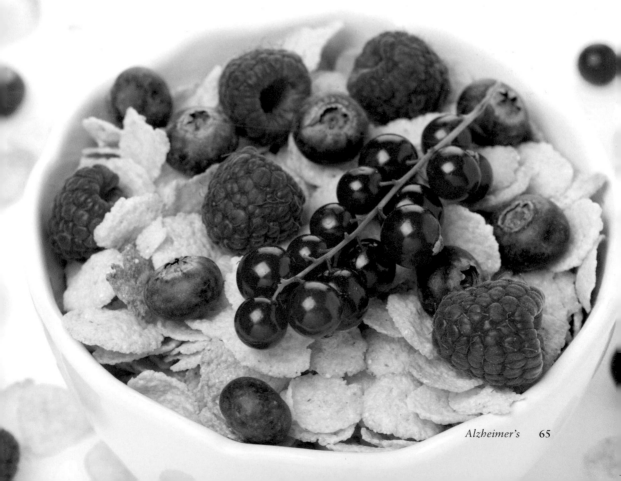

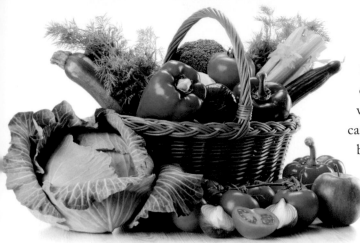

Whole Grains: Oatmeal, oat bran, brown rice, barley, and whole wheat flour are complex carbohydrates that help to stabilize blood glucose levels. Your body digests simple carbohydrates – the kind you find in refined white flour and sugar and loads of processed foods – too quickly, resulting in abrupt energy spikes and plummets. Glucose is the brain's main fuel source, so it is important to stick with foods that contain whole grains to keep glucose in steady supply and maintain your concentration.

Fresh Veggies: Pile your plate with leafy green and cruciferous vegetables like kale, cabbage, cauliflower and brussels sprouts. Eat plenty of salads and stir-fries and vegetable side dishes. Vegetables are full of antioxidants, vitamin C, and plant compounds called carotenoids. Carotenoids are plant pigments and contain vitamin A, a powerful antioxidant that is particularly helpful is removing toxic free-radicals from the brain.

Avocados, Oils, Nuts, and Seeds: Although vitamin E can be consumed as a supplement, studies show that when vitamin E is obtained through food, a person can lower their risk for Alzheimer's by up to 67%. Good sources of vitamin E are avocados, almonds, hazelnuts, pistachios, pecans, walnuts, sunflower, pumpkin, and sesame seeds, and canola oil. Cooked butternut squash, pumpkin, and fresh spinach are also good food sources of vitamin E.

Water: Drinking water helps you (and your brain) stay hydrated and healthy. A study published in the journal *Frontiers in Human Neuroscience* says that people who drink water to quench thirst perform better on mental tests. Researchers from the University of East London and the University of Westminster in the United Kingdom had participants complete a number of mental tests – an experiment on a "thirsty" group showed that performance was improved once the thirst was relieved. Separate research has found that failing to drink enough water can shrink the brain's grey matter, making it harder to think.

EAT THE RAINBOW!

Choosing fruits and vegetables with vibrant colors ensures that they are packed with fiber, vitamins, and minerals. The more color on your plate, the more healthful it is!

✔ **Red:** bell peppers, cherries, cranberries, onions, red beets, strawberries, tomatoes, watermelon

✔ **Blue and Purple:** blackberries, blueberries, grapes, plums, purple cabbage, purple carrots, purple potatoes

✔ **Orange and Yellow:** apricots, bananas, carrots, mangoes, oranges, peaches, squash, sweet potatoes

✔ **Green:** avocado, broccoli, cabbage, cucumber, dark lettuce, grapes, honeydew, kale, kiwi, spinach, zucchini

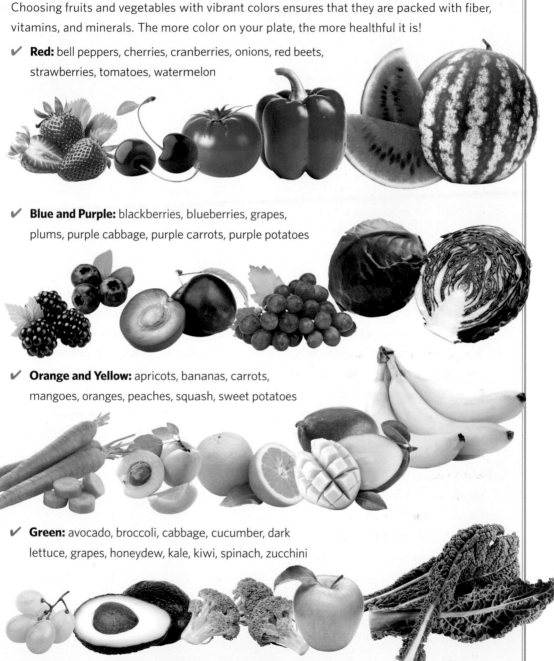

Chocolate Keeps the Brain Sharp in Old Age

A study led by neurologist Farzaneh A. Sorond at Brigham and Women's Hospital in Boston, Massachusetts and published in the journal *Neurology* suggests that eating chocolate may help improve brain health and thinking skills in the elderly. Researchers tested two groups: one with reduced blood flow to the brain and neuron damage, and another control group with far less neuron damage and better blood flow.

The participants in the study who had reduced blood flow initially performed poorly on a memory and reasoning test, but after drinking two cups of cocoa every day for a month, they showed an improvement in blood flow as well as improved reaction times to cognitive tasks. The test results showed a correlation between blood flow to the brain and cognitive function, relating to earlier findings that people with high blood pressure and other cardiovascular conditions were prone to developing dementia.

While consuming chocolate and chocolate-related products might be good for the brain, it is important to remember that it can also result in weight gain. The amounts of cocoa the study participants drank were offset by dietary constraints and exercise. Eating dark chocolate (at least 70% cacao), which is lower in fat and sugar than milk chocolate, is your best option for avoiding unwanted consequences. Dark chocolate has cardiovascular benefits, can help to counteract insulin resistance, and is high in antioxidants. Bonus: studies show that consuming dark chocolate in moderation coupled with regular exercise actually boosts weight loss.

Coffee and Green Tea Are Protective Factors for Alzheimer's

Coffee

Several studies have been conducted that show how consumption of caffeine acts as a protective factor for Alzheimer's disease by decreasing the production of abnormal beta-amyloid. But more recently, a study by researchers at the University of South Florida published in the *Journal of Alzheimer's Disease* asserts that specifically caffeinated coffee increases the blood levels of a growth factor called GCSF – a substance in low supply in Alzheimer's patients.

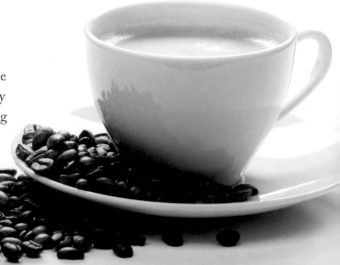

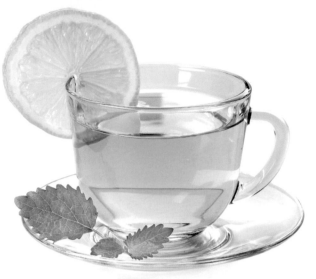

Conducting an animal study, the researchers demonstrated that caffeinated coffee, not caffeine alone, increases GCSF, noting that an as-yet-unidentified component in coffee interacts with the caffeine to produce this effect.

GCSF levels in the blood supply are important because they enhance memory by removing beta-amyloid and increasing the production of neurons and the connections between them. Scientists say that regularly consuming 4-5 cups of coffee per day (drip coffee – not frothy, calorie-laden concoctions) is necessary to reduce your risk for and delay the onset of Alzheimer's.

Coffee keeps your brain sharp, is an excellent antioxidant, elevates mood, and reduces your risk for type-2 diabetes.

Consume moderate amounts of coffee daily only if you have not been otherwise restricted from drinking coffee or other caffeinated beverages due to pre-existing health concerns.

Green Tea

Several studies have been published recently that point to green tea's potential as a potent protective factor for Alzheimer's disease. Specifically, two components of green tea – resveratrol and EGCG – have been shown to protect the brain against deterioration. EGCG and resveratrol are polyphenols, plant chemicals that work as antioxidants to protect the cells in your body from free-radical damage.

Studies have shown that the consumption of green tea can be effective in breaking down and clearing out excess accumulation of beta-amyloid proteins in the brain, improving memory function in study participants. Consuming green tea can also increase neurogenesis – the production of brain cells.

One study also showed that the more green tea a subject consumed, the higher the increase in brain activity, which highlights a straightforward cause-and-effect relationship between drinking green tea and improving brain function.

Try drinking green tea as often as possible. It is relatively inexpensive and makes a great substitute for sugary soft drinks and juice blends that are high in calories and simple carbs but low on nutrients.

The Yuzu – A Citrus Super-fruit

Common citrus fruits like oranges, lemons, tangerines, and grapefruit all contain high amounts of the antioxidant vitamin C, but a fruit native to China and cultivated in Japan and Korea called the yuzu has powerful protective properties that scientists have begun tapping into. Animal studies have shown that its consumption prevents neurodegenerative damage and insulin resistance that would otherwise lead to Alzheimer's.

Yuzu has three times the vitamin C of lemon, and its main weapon against Alzheimer's is flavonoids – bioactive compounds that cross the blood-brain barrier and act as anti-inflammatory and antioxidant agents. By reducing inflammation and oxidative stress in the brain, flavonoids also reverse insulin resistance in the brain, which results from an accumulation of beta-amyloid plaques, one of the hallmarks of Alzheimer's.

Yuzu is a delicate fruit and is not easy to find whole in supermarkets, but chefs and juice makers have begun featuring its complex floral lime flavor in recipes and bottling it for consumers to enjoy. Look for it in sauces, syrups, sorbets, and even as a component of mixed drinks.

Food Precautions

The following is a list of foods and substances that have been linked to Alzheimer's disease, heart disease, or diabetes in some way. While it might not be realistic – or even advisable in some cases – to stop eating all of the following foods, it is good to be aware of the risks associated with them so that you can make more informed dietary choices, enjoying some foods in moderation while finding more healthful alternatives for others.

Acid Load – Fruits and vegetables are not the enemy: Acid load, or excess acid, can spark complications in the metabolic system that reduce the body's ability to regulate its insulin levels, leading to diabetes. A common misconception is that fruits or other foods high in citric acid trigger the stomach acids linked to diabetes. In fact, the opposite is true. Most fruits and vegetables actually form alkaline precursors in the stomach that neutralize acidity, whereas animal products such as **meat, cheese, and egg yolks** increase dietary acid load. Unless your cholesterol is skyrocketing, don't cut out meat altogether. Instead, cut down on the frequency and portion size of the meats you consume, eat more fish or vegetarian entrees, and try to fill half of your plate with whole fruits and vegetables, leaving ¼ for meat and ¼ for grains or starch.

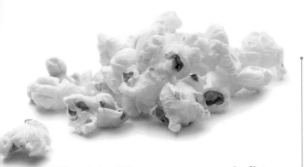

Diacetyl – Microwave popcorn's dirty secret: Diacetyl is a food flavoring used to enhance the taste of butter flavoring in processed foods such as **microwave popcorn, margarine, candy, cultured sour cream, and baked goods**. Diacetyl has been linked in the past to fatal lung disease and more recently to Alzheimer's. Researchers have found that the molecular structure of diacetyl resembles that of a substance that makes beta-amyloid clump together. Diacetyl can penetrate the blood-brain barrier, a layer of cells designed to keep harmful agents from entering the brain. In lab tests, diacetyl has been found toxic to nerve cells by blocking glyoxalase, a protective protein that safeguards neurons.

Instead of resorting to microwave popcorn and its "buttery topping," air pop whole corn kernels and flavor them with your favorite combination of toppings – try cinnamon and sugar, or cracked pepper and parmesan. To make your own "microwave" popcorn, simply pour two tablespoons of popcorn kernels into a brown paper bag, fold the top down and tape it shut. Place the bag upright in the microwave and cook on high for two minutes or until the popping sounds slow down.

Diet Soda – it's not really calorie free: Zero-calorie soft drinks have long been used to cut calories while satisfying people's soda cravings. But more recently, nutritionists and researchers contend that diet soda actually causes people to gain weight because more often than not, they are likely to snack while drinking diet soda, taking on excess calories.

The sweet taste of diet soda signals to your stomach that sugar and calories are entering your system, which triggers hormones that process sugar to prepare for digestion. In other words, you are giving your body the taste of nourishment without any actual nourishment or nutrients to digest. When the calories don't come, the body's metabolism is thrown off because you feel hungrier than you should, so you eat to quell the hunger the diet soda triggered, thus sabotaging good eating habits and gaining weight.

Over time, with regular diet soda consumption, your body could actually stop releasing the hormones that process sugar at the same level or even altogether as a response to this confusion. Studies have linked the regular consumption of diet soda to higher risks for type-2 diabetes, stroke, high blood pressure, heart disease, and metabolic syndrome.

Drink simple filtered water, sparkling water, or even iced coffee whenever possible, and do your best to avoid all soft drinks – the high sugar content in regular soda or sweet tea won't do you any favors.

Nitrites - what are they preserving?

Nitrites are salts used as preservatives to prevent meat from spoiling and becoming contaminated with bacteria. Examples of preserved meats include: **cured meats, such as bacon and hot dogs; fermented meats, such as bologna, salami, corned beef, ham, and sausage; and smoked meats, such as salmon, trout, and chicken**. Nitrites can affect the brain's ability to use glucose by preventing glucose from reaching neurons thus causing neurodegeneration. Nitrites, coupled with an overall high-fat diet, can exacerbate this cell death. Which would you prefer eating – food that won't spoil or food that won't spoil your brain? If you

must, enjoy these nitrite-rich products as occasional treats rather than dietary staples. When packing your daily lunch, try making your sandwich with some leftover roast chicken or turkey, canned tuna, or hummus and veggies instead.

Vegetable Oils - they're not all created equal:

Omega-3 fatty acids are vital nutrients found in olive and canola oils as well as in fish like salmon, mackerel, and sardines. Like omega-3s, omega-6 fatty acids are essential – meaning the body can't make them on its own and needs to obtain them through food – but consuming too many omega-6 fatty acids can result in inflammation. The **omega-6 fatty acids found in corn and safflower oil** oxidize easily in our bodies, leading to the oxidative stress and inflammation that increase heart disease risk, despite the fact that they can reduce cholesterol. Our bodies need omega-6, but it is easy to over-consume because it is found in so many processed foods – even those claiming to be healthy – like **frozen foods, crackers, cereals, and bottled salad dressing**. The best way to limit their consumption is to read food labels, screening for omega-6 sources, and to cook with omega-3-rich oils like canola, soybean, and olive oil. Seek out good sources of omega-6, such as avocados, walnuts, cashews, flax seeds, and coconut that contain linoleic acid, which is vital to your health.

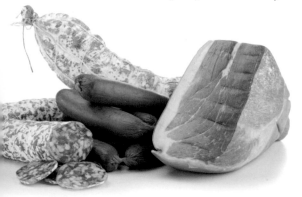

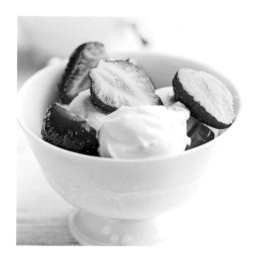

Real Whipped Cream Won't Kill You - Seriously: A dollop of whipped cream contains about 50 calories and under 2 grams of saturated fat, making it a minor indulgence when enjoyed sparingly. **Whipped cream substitutes like Cool Whip and Reddi-wip** contain around the half the calories; however, to achieve this, their ingredients consist of an unhealthy mix of hydrogenated oils, high fructose corn syrup, and chemical additives that give them a virtually infinite shelf life. Guess what's missing? The cream! Real whipped cream, on the other hand, is made from a maximum of three ingredients: heavy cream occasionally paired with a small amount of sugar and/or vanilla extract, with zero additives. It might require a little extra effort to take out your hand mixer and make your own, but real whipped cream beats the convenience and health risks of non-dairy whipped topping every time.

Have a Drink, But Don't Drink to Excess

If you like a cocktail now and then (around one a day) go ahead and enjoy a drink. Alcohol isn't a protective factor for Alzheimer's, but for those people who are already moderate drinkers, it won't necessarily raise your risk. On the other hand, those who binge drink or regularly have four or more drinks at one sitting are much more likely to experience memory problems. Moreover, regular binge drinking can lead to other problems such as high blood pressure and diabetes complications.

As a rule, if you are a moderate drinker, limit yourself to fewer than 14 drinks per week. If you are a binge drinker, try to curb your alcohol consumption or stop drinking all together. And if you have never been a drinker, don't start drinking as a way to stave off Alzheimer's disease. Studies show that starting to drink at an older age could actually raise your risk for memory problems.

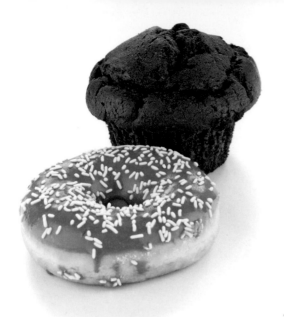

The Snack Food Trap

Many dieticians and nutritionists now advocate eating between meals to manage hunger and avoid binge eating. Snacking, once thought of as a way to pile on unnecessary calories, is now viewed as a way to improve and reinforce healthy eating habits; however, the quality and quantity of your snack is vital to this principle. It is important to choose healthful snacks – ones that are high in lean protein, vitamins, minerals, and dietary fiber but relatively low in calories, trans fats, sugar, and salt.

Not everything that is labeled a snack is suitable for snacking, so refer to the following tips when making your snacking choices.

- Calories matter when snacking. Eat no more than around 100 calories per snack.
- Eat enough to be satisfied without turning a snack into a meal.
- Turn the package over and read the label. The front of the box or bag is often deceiving, claiming that food is "healthy" when it's not.
- Steer clear of foods that contain trans fats and are high in salt and sugar.
- If you can't recognize most of the ingredients listed on the label of your snack, don't eat it.
- Eat "real" food. If your snack can go bad, it's good for you; if it can't, it's not.
- Vending machines typically offer the kinds of high-fat, low-nutrition, processed foods you should avoid.
- Dessert is not a good snack option. Snack cakes, pies, cookies, and donuts are full of unhealthful refined sugars, trans fats, and simple carbohydrates.
- Not only are potato chips and other bagged snack foods salt and fat-laden, but they are some of the easiest foods to binge on without realizing it. Eating two or three ounces (55-85g) of chips will skyrocket you past your 100 calorie limit.
- If they are an overeating trigger for you, remove grain-based snack options from your diet. Refined carbohydrates sabotage weight loss goals.
- A "low fat" label is not a license to overindulge.
- Don't drink soda or "energy" drinks.

Good snack options:

✔ Fruits and vegetables, including: apples, avocados, bananas, brussels sprouts, cantaloupe, carrots, celery with apple butter, dried cherries, dried cranberries, dried figs, grapes, grapefruit, raspberries, tomato with ground pepper and olive oil
✔ Roasted almonds
✔ Plain, low-fat yogurt with honey
✔ Air-popped popcorn (not pre-bagged microwave popcorn)
✔ Sunflower seeds
✔ Dark chocolate
✔ Sardines
✔ Lean turkey breast with Swiss cheese
✔ Cottage cheese
✔ Hummus

Transition to Better Eating Habits

For most people, abruptly switching to a new diet plan isn't realistic, but you cannot use inconvenience as an excuse to avoid changing the way you eat. Good eating habits can be developed over time by introducing one or two small changes to your dining choices incrementally until they become habit. With the variety of healthful, good-tasting, and satisfying foods available in the diet plan suggestions, there is no reason for permanent excuses.

Experiment by making substitutions in your daily menu to discover new favorite foods. If you can stick with it, you will easily transition into a new food lifestyle that no longer causes you to crave those foods you once thought you couldn't live without.

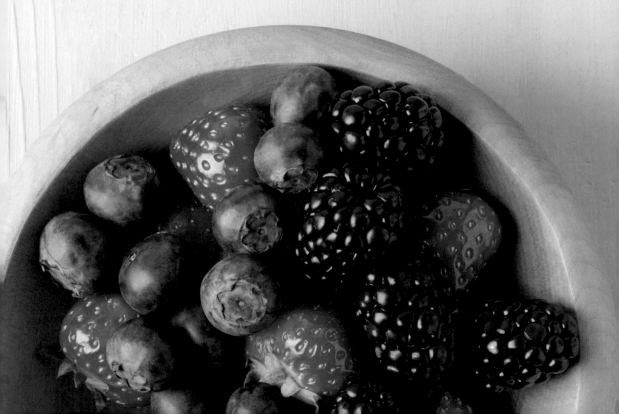

Breakfast

- Have a bowl of oatmeal instead of a sugary processed cereal. Use plain, steel cut oats whenever possible (avoid the instant and flavored varieties) and flavor it with dried fruits such as raisins, cranberries, or acai berries, and some cinnamon.

- It's fine to splurge on bacon or sausage once in a while, but if breakfast meat is a staple for you, cut down on your saturated fat intake by substituting Canadian bacon or veggie sausage as your protein. And always make sure to beware of your nitrite intake.

- Think in "either/or" terms. If you have a piece of cheese with your breakfast, don't also have a bowl full of cereal and milk, adding on extra dairy. If you eat toast, don't also have a huge glass of juice, piling on the carbs.

- Whole fruits and vegetables are best.

- Punches and juice "cocktails" contain far less fruit juice and more sugar than plain, fresh-squeezed juice. Whole fruits and vegetables are an even better choice.

- When grabbing breakfast on the go at your local coffee shop, remember that donuts consist of fried dough and sugar, and muffins are basically mini cakes. Try a cup of yogurt with fruit and granola or a vegetable and fruit smoothie instead – the protein and vitamins will sustain you until lunch without making you feel sluggish.

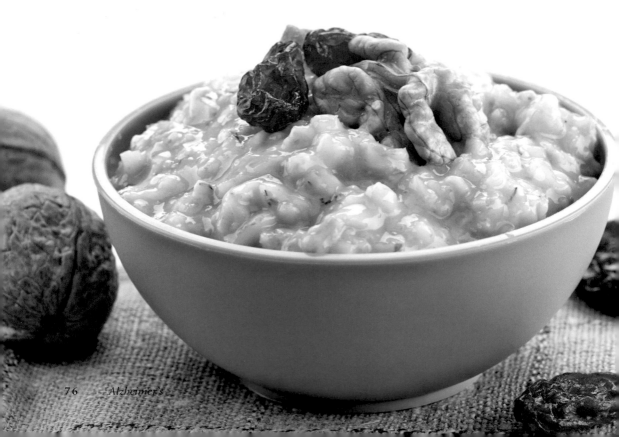

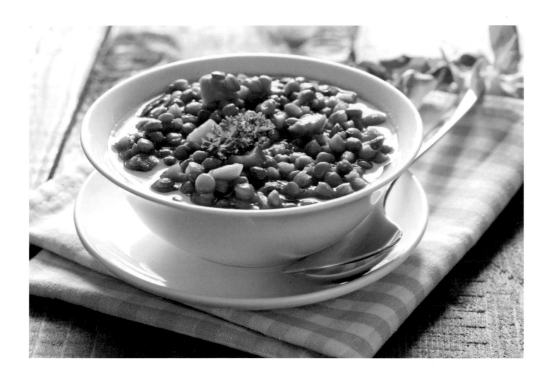

Lunch and Dinner

- Designate days of the week as meat-free. Choose at least one day a week when you go vegetarian, eating no meat or fish during any meal or snack. Designate one or two more days as fish days, leaving three or four days as chicken and meat days. Gradually see if you can invert the proportion of meat days to fish and veggie days, so that you are eventually consuming red meat only three to four times per month.
- Soups and stews made from vegetables and legumes such as lentils, beans, and peas, can be made in large batches to be divided and frozen for easy access in a pinch as a good alternative to the drive through or pizza delivery on a busy evening.
- Lean meats and poultry are best. Choose from: skinless chicken and turkey breast or thigh, filet mignon or New York strip steak trimmed of fat, pork tenderloin, center cut pork loin chops, organ meats, and game meats such as venison, buffalo, duck, ostrich, and rabbit.
- Whenever possible, pack your lunch so that you can control exactly what goes into it.

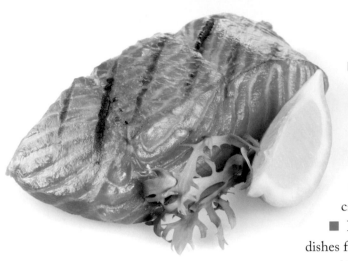

Restaurants

If you eat out frequently, it is important that you develop some guidelines for the kind of food you order until avoiding unwise choices becomes second nature.

- Take advantage of a restaurant's heart-healthy menu suggestions. Today, restaurants are more in tune with people's increasingly health-conscious lifestyles and their menus will often indicate the lower-fat, lower-calorie options.

- Try to stay away from the drive-thru. Fast food restaurants offer some of the most high-calorie, high-fat and high-sodium food with the least nutritional payoff. If you do eat fast food, opt for water instead of soda, order the smallest portion sizes of sandwiches and french fries available, and read the nutritional information for each menu item so that you can make better-informed choices.

- As a rule of thumb, avoid the pasta portion of the menu. Standard semolina pasta is a source of simple carbohydrates and high calories without the corresponding nutritional value and is often served with high-calorie, high-fat sauce.

- If you have a choice in side dishes for your entrée, double up on your vegetable portions – as long as they aren't drenched in creams and cheese sauces.

- If you order steak, avoid the cuts with the highest fat content, like prime rib, porterhouse or rib eye (also known as Delmonico steak, entrecote, or Scotch filet.) Instead, opt for a tenderloin filet, omitting the heavy, creamy sauce accompaniments. Choose the smallest cut that is available – no one needs 32 ounces (900g) of anything to feel full.

- Have a curry. Spices used in Thai and Indian cuisine fight inflammation and might actually help to clear away Alzheimer's-causing protein deposits.

- Good fish choices include wild caught salmon, tuna, mackerel, and sardines, which are all high in omega-3 fatty acid.

- If you order dessert – share it!

- Definitely treat yourself on occasion, but don't turn rich, calorie-laden appetizers and entrees into a standard order.

The Supermarket

- Try to plan meals ahead of time as often as possible. Arm yourself with a strategy and a shopping list when you go to the supermarket to keep from making impulse purchases.

- Shop on a full stomach. You'll be less likely to crave foods that are bad for you or convenient to eat in a hurry to satisfy your hunger.

- Spend most of your time in the fresh produce aisle, followed by the fresh seafood and fresh meat and poultry counters. The less time you spend in aisles with boxed, bagged, and canned goods that can rest on the shelf almost indefinitely, the better. If it spoils easily, don't be afraid to eat it – always in moderation, of course!

- Steer clear of the snack food isle. The chips, pretzels, and other salty-crunchy treats available there are laden with preservatives and unhealthy oils, dyes, and flavorings, and are some of the most highly addictive foods you can eat. The saying is true – you can't have just one chip.

- Read labels. Labels are your best defense against eating harmful ingredients and taking in too many empty calories.

- Swap refined carbohydrates for whole grain food. Buy brown rice instead of white and try whole wheat pasta in your next Italian dish.

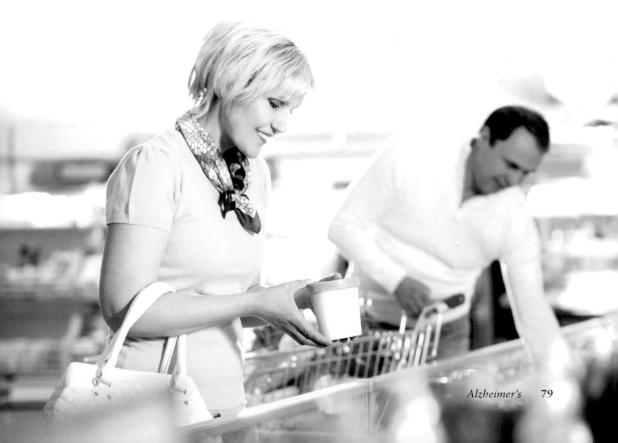

ANTI-OXIDANT RICH FOODS TO ADD TO YOUR SHOPPING LIST

✔ Cruciferous vegetables: broccoli, cauliflower, cabbage, bok choy, and Brussels sprouts

✔ Leafy greens: kale, collard greens, turnip greens, Swiss chard, mustard greens, and spinach

✔ Berries: blueberries, cranberries, raspberries, blackberries, and strawberries

✔ Artichokes

✔ Fresh tomatoes rather than canned. *cooking tomatoes allows your body to absorb the antioxidant lycopene more easily

✔ Orange/yellow-colored fruits: oranges, tangerines, mangoes, peaches, cantaloupe and pineapple

✔ Other fruits: apples, black plums, sweet cherries, and red grapes

✔ Dried fruit without added sugar

✔ Beans: red beans, kidney beans and black beans

✔ Black and green tea

Food Apps for Staying on Track

Turn your smartphone or tablet into a personal dietary aide by downloading one or more of these apps to assist you as you transition to better eating habits.

✔ **Epicurious** – A compilation of recipes from Conde Nast food publications like *Bon Appetit*, *Gourmet*, and *Self* magazines, as well as recipe collections from renowned chefs and cookbooks, Epicurious allows you to search for recipes by keyword and to account for dietary restrictions by excluding undesired ingredients or food groups.

✔ **Food Substitutes** – When you have a recipe that is too high in calories or fat or that contains an ingredient you have to avoid, this app helps you find the best food swaps to suit your cooking. It's also great if you've simply forgotten to pick up a key ingredient at the supermarket and need a substitute in a pinch. (for Android devices)

✔ **Fooducate** – This app uses your smartphone to scan the barcodes of grocery store items and issues them a grade from A – F, based on a food's nutritional content and ingredients, eliminating the guesswork from reading food labels and helping you stick to your healthy eating goals. The premium version includes information relating to gluten and allergies.

✔ **Healthy in a Hurry** – The award-winning magazine *EatingWell* has created an app containing fast, easy, health-conscious recipes with straightforward instructions and nutritional information to help you track what is essential to your dietary needs.

✔ **Healthy Out** – A restaurant guide that matches your dietary and nutrition requirements to the appropriate dishes at local restaurants so that you can stay healthy while eating out.

✔ **MyFitnessPal** – A food tracker that provides nutritional information and calorie counts for thousands of foods. Enter a search term, including food and drink items from famous chain restaurants, or scan the barcodes of foods in your fridge and pantry and indicate the serving size you eat to track an accurate measurement of your total calorie, salt, fat, protein, and carbohydrate intake for the day.

✔ **Substitutions** – Like Food Substitutes, Substitutions is Apple's version of a food substitution app that lets you swap recipe ingredients to address nutrition and allergy concerns. (for Apple devices)

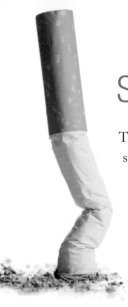

SMOKING AND ALZHEIMER'S

The consequences of smoking have been well-publicized for decades. Inhaling a cigarette's toxic combination of chemicals can lead to heart disease, stroke, chronic bronchitis, and emphysema. It also reduces blood circulation by narrowing arteries and leads to infertility. Smoking causes cancers of the lung, esophagus, larynx, mouth, throat, kidney, bladder, pancreas, stomach, and cervix.

More recently, researchers have found a link between smoking and an increased risk for Alzheimer's and dementia. A study led by Dr. Claudio Soto of the University of Texas Health Science Center in Houston concluded that exposure to cigarette smoke caused increased disease abnormalities in the brains of mice, pointing to smoking as a potential environmental risk factor for Alzheimer's disease. The study found that the mice who were exposed to cigarette smoke displayed signs of neuroinflammation as well as a buildup of amyloid plaques and tau proteins.

If you are a smoker, add Alzheimer's to the list of diseases that quitting might prevent.

Five Steps for Preparing to Quit

STEP 1 — SET A QUIT DATE

Give yourself a two week window to quit. Pick a day within those two weeks and determine to make it the last day you put a cigarette to your mouth. Make sure to choose a day when you will be relatively stress-free and not very busy.

STEP 2 — TELL OTHERS ABOUT YOUR PLAN TO QUIT

Hold yourself accountable by having others hold you accountable. Telling other people you love and respect of your intention to quit means that you will be more likely to stick to your plan, lest you let them down. Your loved ones will also want to help you through the tough times, making it a little easier for you to succeed.

✔ Try partnering up with a friend who also wants to quit so that you can help one another.

✔ Take part in smoke-free activities with friends and family to pass the time.

✔ Tell friends to hold you to your promise to quit and to keep you from smoking at all costs when they are around you.

✔ Ask loved ones to check in on you during your journey and ask them to be patient on days when you are in a bad mood.

STEP 3
PLAN FOR CHALLENGES ALONG THE WAY

Quitting smoking isn't an easy proposition for most people, so be prepared to face withdrawal symptoms, nagging cravings, and uncomfortable feelings during the process. During the first few weeks you will most likely experience some of the following:

■ Depression
■ Sleeplessness
■ Cranky, frustrated mood
■ Nervousness and restlessness
■ Anger
■ Clouded thoughts

Don't resist these emotions, they are a natural part of quitting. Allow yourself to feel your feelings and remember that they will pass. Talk to someone about your experience or find a way to distract yourself until they pass – they are only temporary.

STEP 4
REMOVE CIGARETTES FROM YOUR ENVIRONMENT

Prepare yourself for quitting day by removing any trace of cigarettes and smoking paraphernalia like lighters and ashtrays from your environment. Throw away the cigarettes you keep at home, work, and in your car, and make sure to root out and discard any secret stashes you have tucked away so that you are not tempted to reach for them in a moment of weakness. If possible, remove the trace scent of smoking from your environment as well. Smoke tends to linger in fabrics like carpet and drapery, as well as in your car.

STEP 5
DON'T USE OTHER TOBACCO PRODUCTS AS A SUBSTITUTE FOR CIGARETTES

All tobacco products are dangerous to your health, so substituting pipes, cigars, chewing tobacco, or clove cigarettes for regular cigarettes is no solution. Instead, talk to your doctor or pharmacist about your options for quitting aids such as nicotine patches or gum.

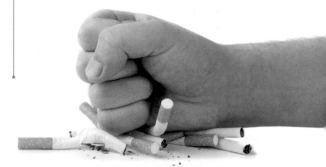

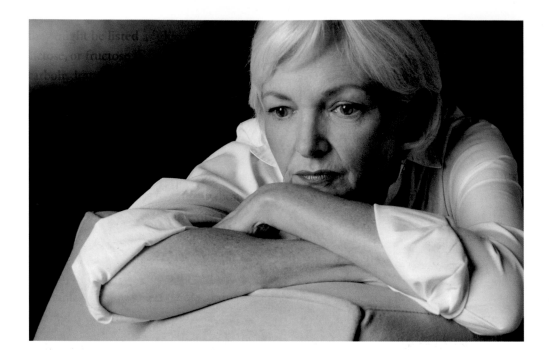

How to Respond to Triggers and Handle Cravings

Smokers develop routines and rituals, such as stepping out for a cigarette during a work break, or smoking after a meal, that become ingrained in their daily lives, so learning how to identify triggers and quell cravings is essential to successfully kicking the habit.

Common triggers include:
✔ Stress
✔ Feeling down
✔ Talking on the phone
✔ Driving
✔ Drinking alcohol
✔ Having coffee
✔ Loneliness

You have to identify your personal triggers so that you can handle cravings. When you are triggered to smoke, recognize the trigger and then try to resist the urge to light up. It might be tough at first, but remember that cravings typically last only 5-10 minutes before they pass. To pass the time, try the following:

- **Phone or text a friend or relative.** Use the communication as a distraction. If no one is available to chat, call a smoking hotline to talk to an expert about what you are experiencing.
- **Have something on hand to do to pass the time.** Arm yourself with a portable distraction that you can carry with you when the urge to smoke

strikes. Read a magazine, listen to your music player, or play a game on your phone. When you focus your attention away from the smoking, you'll see that your craving has passed before you know it.

- **Take a walk, weather and time permitting.** If you're stuck indoors or at work, go up and down the stairs several times. Not only will your craving pass, but you'll be performing some good cardio work in the process.

- **Go to a place where smoking is prohibited** – most public places no longer allow smoking. Find a store, library, movie theater, museum, or any place where you would like to pass the time while being forced not to smoke.

- **Do the math.** Remind yourself how much money you are saving by no longer purchasing expensive packs of cigarettes.

- **Keep your mouth busy** – chew some gum or suck on a lollipop.

- **Breathe deeply.** Inhale through your nose and exhale through your mouth. Doing this ten times should do the trick, with the added benefit of reducing your stress level in the process.

- **Do not bargain with yourself** by rationalizing that you'll only smoke three puffs or half a cigarette. Not smoking is the only option if you're serious about quitting.

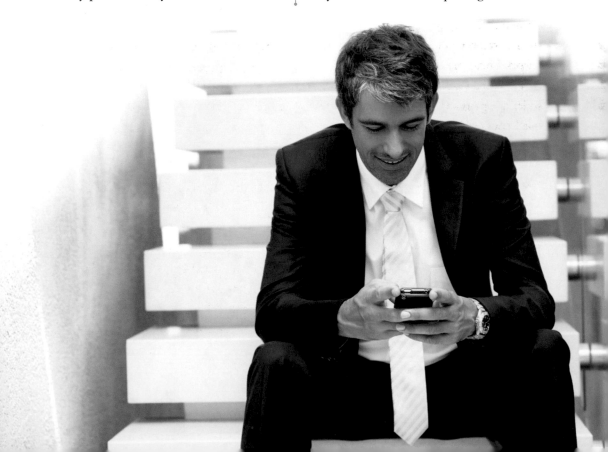

The Stress Link

Stress is a major trigger for smoking, and quitting smoking results in stress, so what can you do to break the cycle, curb stress, and stay committed to being smoke-free?

Since stress is a part of life, learning to identify what causes you stress and how to minimize or deal with it is a key part of the quitting process. It is important that you identify your own stress triggers and seek out ways to deal with them that work best for you.

✔ **Exercise.** Exercising releases endorphins – feel-good neurotransmitters that help us experience pleasure, improve our mood, and reduce stress.
✔ **Breathe.** Take several controlled breaths, inhaling through your nose and exhaling through your mouth, and allow your body to relax.
✔ **Locate parts of your body that feel tension and find ways to alleviate it.** Your body can tighten up in stressful moments or after prolonged stress, causing pain and discomfort. Try stretching or massaging with ointment to ease the tension.
✔ **Remove yourself from stressful situations.** You can't run from stress, but it's okay to step away momentarily when you need a breather. Taking a five-minute break from the work piling up on your desk allows you to clear your head and push on. But don't use those five minutes for smoking. Have a healthy snack, chat with a friend or coworker, or take a quick walk.
✔ **Practice positive visualization.** Close your eyes for a moment and think of something that makes you happy – a dream vacation destination, social plans you've made, or your cozy bed. Take a few minutes to imagine yourself being in that location and allow yourself to experience the pleasure you associate with it.
✔ **Face your stress head on.** If there is something (or someone) causing you stress and you can do something about it, face your fear and confront the problem.
✔ **Focus on the present.** Sometimes when we try to anticipate future events or outcomes, we wind up imagining the most unrealistic worst-case scenarios, creating anxiety and losing focus on what's in front of us. Try to take your life – and your quitting journey – one day, one hour, one moment at a time.

Smoking and Weight Control

An unintended consequence of quitting might be weight gain, and previous sections of this book have already highlighted how being overweight is a risk factor for Alzheimer's. But don't

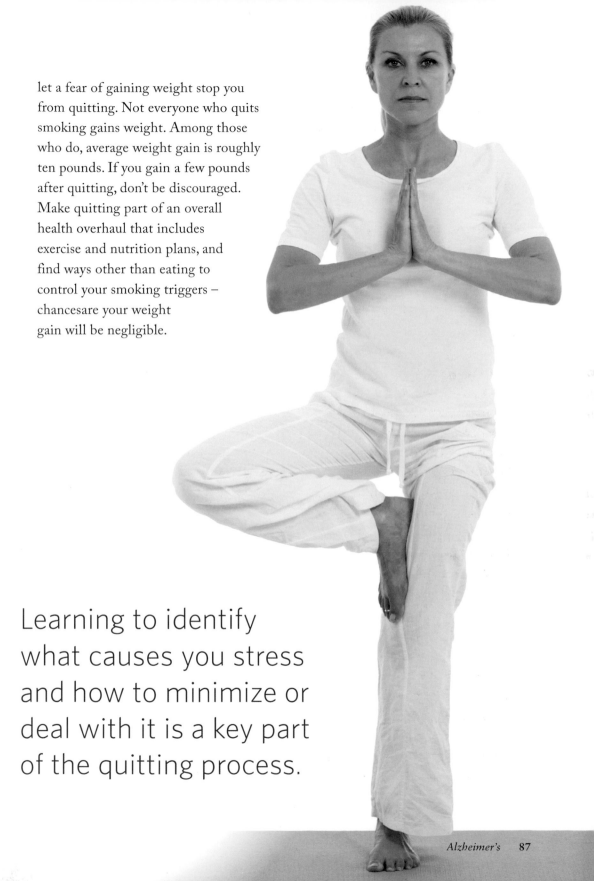

let a fear of gaining weight stop you from quitting. Not everyone who quits smoking gains weight. Among those who do, average weight gain is roughly ten pounds. If you gain a few pounds after quitting, don't be discouraged. Make quitting part of an overall health overhaul that includes exercise and nutrition plans, and find ways other than eating to control your smoking triggers – chancesare your weight gain will be negligible.

Learning to identify what causes you stress and how to minimize or deal with it is a key part of the quitting process.

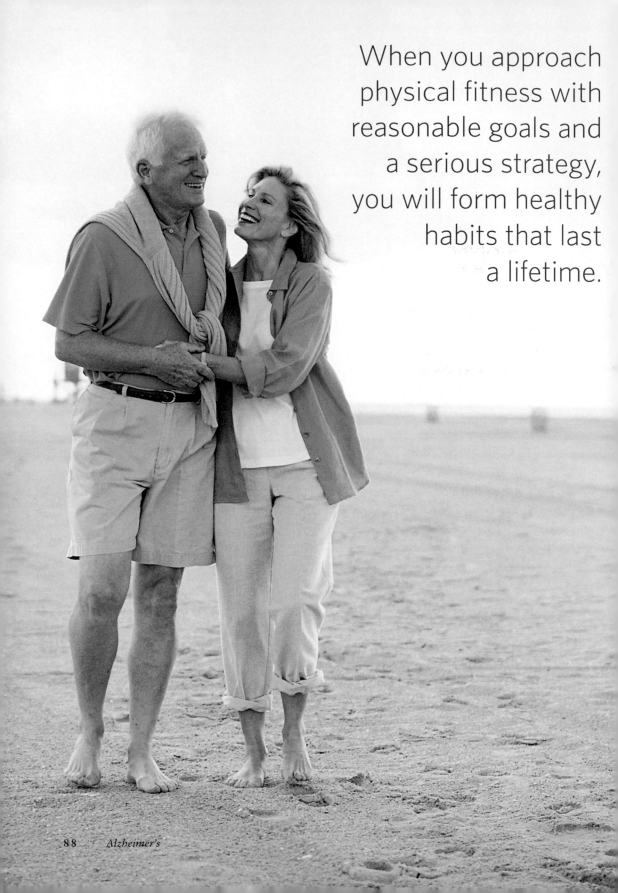

When you approach physical fitness with reasonable goals and a serious strategy, you will form healthy habits that last a lifetime.

PHYSICAL FITNESS

Why is Physical Fitness Important?

A sedentary lifestyle – one that involves little to no regular exercise and where most time is spent sitting or lying down – is a major contributing factor to lifestyle diseases and conditions like high blood pressure, high cholesterol, coronary artery disease, and type-2 diabetes.

Regular physical activity is a protective factor for these diseases, and recent studies show that it can safeguard against Alzheimer's disease as well – the Alzheimer's Association recommends at least 30 minutes of physical activity per day.

An exercise plan that incorporates aerobic workouts, as well as strength, flexibility, and balance training is beneficial to nearly everyone, but you must consider your fitness goals and your level of experience when designing your exercise program. If you are a beginner, registering for a grueling fitness course at the gym or attempting a long distance run will most likely prove too difficult and might discourage you from exercising all together. It could even lead to physical injury or serious health complications. But when you approach physical fitness with reasonable goals and a serious strategy, you will form healthy habits that last a lifetime.

Exercise and Brain Health

The physical benefits of regular exercise are evident, from weight loss and increased muscle tone to improved cardiovascular health. But another reason to get moving is that physical health promotes brain health. Studies show that exercise provides a wide range of brain benefits.

One reason for this is that physical exercise actually requires the brain to do a lot of work. Your brain has to coordinate complex movements when you exercise, so it's not only your muscles getting a workout. Complicated activities like playing tennis or taking dance lessons increase the level of brain chemicals called growth factors, which help to form neurons and establish new connections between them that improve learning. Complicated activities also improve your capacity to learn by enhancing your attention and concentration skills.

Aerobic training for at least 30 minutes helps to reduce stress by raising the level of brain chemicals like serotonin, dopamine, and norepinephrine that promote relaxation. It can also reroute blood flow away from areas of the brain that cause you to relive stressful situations, making you less likely to think about them repeatedly.

Exercise can be an effective antidepressant because it appears to stimulate the growth of neurons in certain regions of the brain damaged by depression. When you exercise, your body releases chemicals called endorphins. In addition to reducing your perception of pain, endorphins trigger a feeling of euphoria that promotes a positive, energizing outlook on life.

Setting Exercise Goals

Particularly for beginners, it is important to set realistic goals that you can build up over time to avoid overexertion and stay motivated.

✔ Aim for 30 minutes of physical activity a day at first, alternating between strength training and aerobic exercise.

✔ Set yourself up for success. Achieve your ultimate goal in small increments. Once your original goal becomes routine, set your next goal a little higher. If you continue to repeat this process, you'll soon be achieving what once seemed impossible.

✔ As you gain strength and endurance, increase the amount of time you exercise each day and attempt more rigorous activity, like a fitness class, if you can.

✔ If you are struggling, start out slowly, exercising for five minutes a day. Each week, add on five minutes to your daily workout until you've worked your way up to 30 minutes of a particular activity.

✔ Don't be discouraged. If physical limitations restrict your exercise goals to a level below what has been recommended, even five minutes of movement will get your blood flowing a little better. If you are able, exercise for five minutes at a time a few times per day to reach a 15-30 minute per day goal.

✔ If you miss a day of exercise, pick up your workouts again the next day and keep on going. If you find you're skipping a lot of work outs, try adding variety to your exercise routine to stay motivated.

✔ Feel proud that you have made the decision to change your habits in order to improve your quality of life. You've earned it.

* Always speak to your doctor before beginning any exercise program. Ask your doctor about taking a stress test to help you establish safe limits for your aerobic and strength training routines. If you have a chronic condition like diabetes or heart disease, make sure to take your doctor's precautions under advisement so that you stay safe as you exercise.

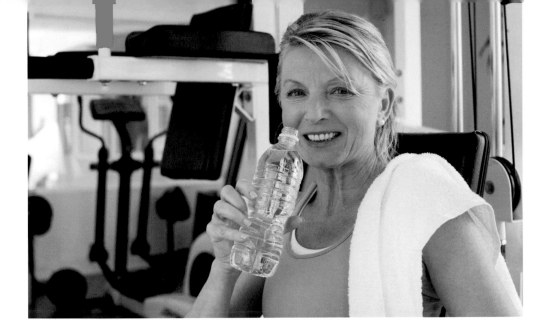

What Kind of Exercise Should I do?

Your exercise routine should include four basic kinds of exercise: **aerobic exercise**, **strength training**, **balance training**, and **stretching**.

AEROBIC EXERCISE

1. Exercises large muscle groups repetitively for a sustained amount of time
2. Raises your heart rate
3. Improves endurance
4. Helps to remove waste and toxins from your body
5. Benefits everyone, no matter their age, weight, or athletic ability.

Aerobic fitness, also called cardio or endurance exercise, is sustained activity that moves large muscle groups, causing you to breathe more deeply and raising your heart rate. The activity must be sustained for a period of time, without stopping and starting, to obtain maximum benefit.

During aerobic activity, your heart beats faster, widening your capillaries (small blood vessels) so that your blood can deliver more oxygen to your muscles and carry away waste products like carbon dioxide and lactic acid. The more regularly you take part in aerobic exercise, the more efficiently your heart, lungs, and blood vessels transport oxygen throughout your body, making routine physical activity much easier. Aerobic exercise should be performed for 30-60 minutes, three to five days per week, so make sure to select activities you enjoy doing for an extended period of time.

Examples of Aerobic Exercise

✔ **Walking** is the most basic aerobic activity and requires no special equipment or location. It is a good first step for anyone who is new to exercising or for whom more intense activities are prohibitive. You can use a treadmill, walk around an indoor or outdoor track, or walk in your neighborhood or local park. The important thing to keep in mind is to set a pace that increases your heart rate, walking with purpose and vigor, to the extent that your physical condition allows.

✔ **Cycling** can be done on a regular or stationary bicycle, which makes it an ideal exercise for rain or shine. It is a good aerobic exercise choice for people with arthritis or other orthopedic problems who can't walk for extended periods of time. It is also a good choice for those individuals who are 50 pounds or more overweight because it helps the heart without putting excess strain on joints like walking or running can.

✔ **Exercise Machines** such as rowing or ski machines, stair climbers, and ellipticals are good options for

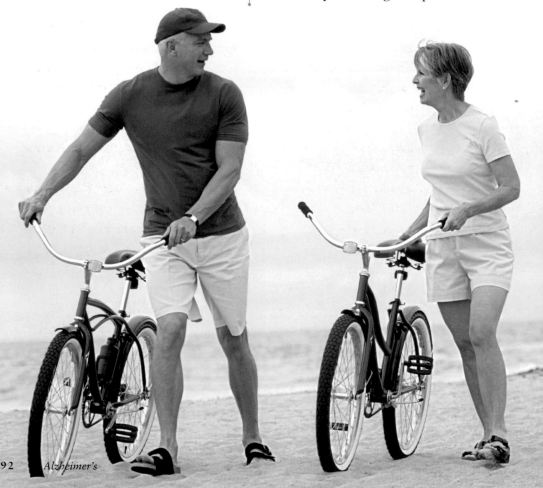

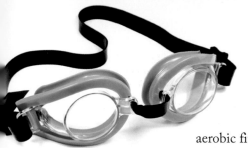

aerobic fitness at the gym, allowing you to increase your pace and intensity over time as your fitness and endurance improve. Try out various machines to figure out which is right for you based on your interest and fitness level, also keeping in mind any joint problems you don't want to exacerbate.

✔ **Swimming** is an excellent, joint-friendly cardiovascular exercise, provided that you are experienced and fit enough to sustain the required intensity to give your heart and muscles a 30-60 minute workout. If you are not a strong swimmer, or if your doctor has ruled out swimming as an exercise option for you, aqua fitness or aqua aerobics are a good alternative for cardio activity that is gentle on the joints.

✔ **Aerobic Fitness Classes** at your local gym are a great way to get in a sustained 30-60 minutes of cardio with the added benefit of an instructor to guide you and hold you accountable. Such classes vary in style and intensity, so talk to someone at the gym to figure out which class is right for you. If you are a beginner, you need to find a class that works with your fitness level and health concerns. Pushing too hard too fast can result in injury or other health consequences.

Walking – A Simple, Highly Beneficial Aerobic Activity

Walking is an uncomplicated, affordable exercise that helps you maintain a healthy weight, strengthens your bones, and lifts your mood. Walking, strength training, and stretching after exercising, combined with a sensible diet, are the basics of achieving and maintaining good physical health.

Technique

To achieve maximum benefit from your walk, you have to concentrate on your stride and body position, turning a leisurely stroll into a fitness walk of purposeful movement.

- Keep your head up and look forward, not at the ground
- Loosen your neck, back, and shoulders for better range of motion.
- Swing your arms freely, with elbows slightly bent if you wish.
- Stand up straight. Do not arch your back forward or backward.
- Tighten your stomach muscles slightly to support your back and remain upright.
- Roll your foot from heel to toe with each stride. Do not drag your feet.

Routine

Keep a consistent walking routine to avoid risk of injury.

✔ Wear shoes with proper arch support for your foot. Not all sneakers or walking shoes are suitable for every foot, so make sure to choose a shoe that supports your foot while keeping it comfortable and pain-free.

✔ When walking outdoors in the dark, wear bright clothing and reflectors so that you are visible to oncoming traffic.

✔ Avoid paths that can easily trip you up. Stay away from courses that have uneven turf or cracked sidewalks and pavement.

✔ Make sure to warm up and cool down. Before setting out on your course or beginning a treadmill routine, walk in place or at a slow pace on the treadmill for five to ten minutes to warm up your muscles. Repeat the process when your course is finished to help your muscles cool down.

✔ Gently stretching your muscles after you cool down is preferable, but if you stretch before your walk make sure to warm up first.

Using a Pedometer

A pedometer is a device that tallies the steps you take by sensing your movement. It counts steps for any step-like activity, such as walking, running, climbing stairs, and even cross country skiing. If you wear a pedometer all day long, it will count the steps you take during your day at the office or while you complete your daily chores.

Tracking your progress can be a great motivational tool. When you set realistic goals for yourself, you keep exercise interesting and set yourself up for success. Keeping a record of how many steps you take, the distance you walk, and the amount of time it takes can serve as a source of inspiration to go even farther.

You can use a pedometer to provide feedback about your walking or jogging routine. When you begin walking or jogging, take note of how many steps you take during your normal route. Once you know the number of steps you take on an average run or walk, set some short term activity goals. For instance, if your normal walk takes about 1,500 steps, set a goal of adding 500 steps per walk. When you've achieved the extra steps, push yourself to add another 500 steps, and so on. Short term goals like these are the building blocks of your overall fitness activity goals.

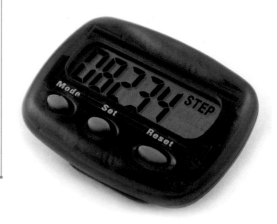

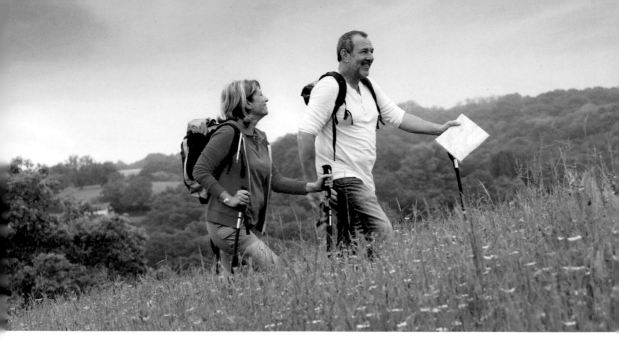

Pioneering Study Shows that Brisk Walking is Most Beneficial

Intensity matters when people walk for health. A study based on new analysis of the National Walkers' and Runners' Health Studies shows that brisk walking produces the equivalent health benefits of running.

Participants in the original runner's and walkers' studies, ranging in age from 18 to 80, reported their height, weight, diet, and the miles per week they spent walking or running for six years. During that time, researchers tracked participants' health problems and concluded that the key to the participants' improved cardiovascular health was the number of calories they burned when exercising rather than the specific activity – running or walking – each participant chose to do regularly. This led researchers to conclude that walking could be just as beneficial to your health as running.

More recently, further research conducted by statistician Dr. Paul T. Williams of the Lawrence Berkeley National Laboratory has revealed that the pace of walking affects the extent of those health benefits. Williams analyzed data from nearly 39,000 walkers who participated in the original study, placing them in four categories according to walking pace. He discovered that the walkers in the slowest two categories, averaging between 20-24 minutes per mile, experienced the least health benefits.

Based on his observations, Dr. Williams recommends walking between 13.5 minutes per mile – on the cusp of jogging – to 17 minutes per mile for maximum calorie burn and health benefit, barring any underlying health conditions that prevent you from keeping such a rigorous pace.

Measuring Your Pace

Measuring your walking speed is key to managing your pace and garnering the most health benefits possible for your efforts. To measure your pace, find a 400-meter track – your local public high school, gymnasium, or park are good options – and using a stopwatch, time yourself walking at your normal speed. If one lap of the track takes you 6 minutes or more, your pace is 24 minutes per mile or slower. If you are strained when attempting to walk at a faster pace than 6 minutes per lap, you should consult your doctor to root out possible underlying health issues that are holding you back.

Otherwise, the best way to improve your walking is to ramp up the pace gradually. The more you walk, the more your stamina builds. Time yourself periodically to see how much you have improved. According to Dr. Williams, the walkers in category 3 of his study moved only around a minute faster per mile than the slowest group but still saw significantly more benefits at their pace compared to the 24 minute group, so any improvement upon your initial time has positive consequences.

Strength training

As aerobic training strengthens your heart, strength training builds the muscles in your arms, legs, and core. When you strength train, you are breaking down muscle tissue so that your body will heal and rebuild the muscle back stronger. Sometimes called weight training, strength training involves repetitive muscle contraction to improve muscle strength, endurance, and bone strength. Typical equipment used for strength training includes weight machines, free weights, and resistance bands, but your own body weight can provide resistance during exercises such as pushups, abdominal crunches, leg lunges, and squats.

STRENGTH TRAINING

1. Increases bone density
2. Helps control weight
3. Boosts stamina and balance
4. Helps reduce the symptoms of chronic conditions such as back pain, arthritis, heart disease, and diabetes
5. Sharpens focus and attention span in older adults

Strength training has a multitude of benefits. It can help stave off age-related muscle loss and osteoporosis, and it can protect you from diabetes and heart disease by increasing your body's ability to use insulin to help process glucose. During the course of a weight loss program, strength training helps you build the lean muscle mass that continues to burn calories in periods of non-activity.

Muscle mass naturally diminishes with age. If you do not incorporate strength training into your fitness regimen, your lean muscle will be gradually replaced by fat. Fat tissue occupies more space under the skin than muscle, so even though you might weigh the same, you will look bulkier and feel more sluggish. Moreover, muscle tissue requires more calories for maintenance than fat tissue, so strength training helps you to maintain your ideal body weight and look leaner – as long as you are eating healthy calories.

Over time, you will see significant changes to your lean muscle mass if you incorporate just two to three 20-30-minute weight training sessions per week into your exercise routine.

STRENGTH TRAINING TIPS

✔ **Aim for tone not bulk:** When you use weight resistance, you build lean muscle over time, and unlike body building, your goal is not to bulk up but to strength and tone.

✔ **Seek help:** If you are new to weight training, the best thing to do is seek the help of a professional who can give you advice on proper form and technique and who can teach you about the various machines and free weights available to you at the gym.

✔ **Start slowly:** In the beginning you might find that you are able to lift only a few pounds at a time, but if you keep at it, you'll see that your body adapts quickly.

✔ **Do one set of repetitions:** A repetition or "rep" is a single cycle of movement through a strength training exercise, lifting the weight and returning to a resting position in a controlled manner. Choose a weight that allows you to do a set of 8-10 reps. If doing 8-10 reps is too easy, the weight is too light. If you struggle to do 8-10 reps, the weight is too heavy and you risk injury. Once you reach a point when you can do 12 reps of a weight comfortably, increase the weight.

✔ **Rest in between workouts:** Strength training works by tearing down muscle and building it back up again, so you need to give your body time to heal. Rest at least one full day before working the same muscle group again. You might achieve this by focusing on a different muscle group each day you strength train or by alternating your strength training and aerobic fitness routines day by day.

✔ **If you are unable to go to a gym to use equipment, try doing pushups and lunges at home.** For relatively little money, you can purchase a strength training video that can guide you in your at-home workout. You can also create makeshift free weights out of gallon jugs and soda cans or purchase inexpensive resistance bands.

Strengthening Your Core

When you incorporate strength training into your exercise routine, don't neglect your core, also called your torso. When you exercise the major muscles of your torso – in your pelvis, lower back, hips, and abdomen – you condition your body to have better posture, balance, and stability. Weak core muscles lead to lower back pain, poor posture, and muscle injuries. Most activities, whether on the athletic field or in the home, require a strong core. You're not gunning for six-pack abs, just an abdomen and back that is are strong enough to help you put away the groceries, lift your grandchild, or take that golf swing without strain or instability. Core exercise are uncomplicated and require no special equipment.

Simple core exercise include:

✔ Abdominal crunches and sit ups
✔ Arm sweeps
✔ Planking
✔ Hip lifts
✔ Wall sits
✔ Single and dual leg bridges

Balance Training

Your sense of balance can deteriorate over time, which can lead to falls and fractures. Older adults in particular should include some form of balance training in their exercise routine to reduce the risk for injury due to falls. Shaky balance can discourage you from exercising or moving in general, which can lead to a downward health spiral.

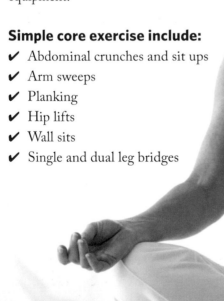

Any activity that keeps you on your feet and moving can help you to maintain good balance, and weight training, which strengthens muscles, increases stability as well; however, incorporating a specific activity that improves your stability into your overall exercise routine is a good idea.

Activities that incorporate balance training include:

✔ Core exercises like sit ups.
✔ Simple movements such as balancing on one leg or walking on a straight line by placing one foot directly in front of the other
✔ Tai Chi – a Chinese system of slow, meditative exercise designed to promote relaxation, balance, and overall health
✔ Yoga – a Hindu discipline that incorporates breath control and specific body postures to promote relaxation, balance, and overall health
✔ Dance – studies show that regular dance lessons improve balance and endurance
✔ Sitting or standing on a balance pillow
✔ Using a balance board
✔ Stability ball or half-ball exercises

If you have never used stability equipment, it is important that you consult with a fitness trainer or physical therapist to prevent injury.

Stretching

1. Improves athletic performance
2. Increases blood flow to muscles
3. Increases range of motion
4. Decreases risk for injury

Don't let stretching take a back seat in your exercise routine. Stretching is key to improving your flexibility and preventing exercise related injury. In turn, improved flexibility allows you to get more benefit out of the exercise you do by increasing your range of motion and increasing blood flow to your muscles.

After you exercise, your muscles are warm and more receptive to stretching, but stretching can be done at any time – before or after exercise or as its own activity. And practices such as yoga and tai chi incorporate stretching into their systems.

Make sure you stretch safely and effectively. And don't consider stretching a simple warm up to exercise – you could actually hurt yourself by stretching cold muscles. Be kind to your muscles by taking 10 minutes before stretching to do a low-intensity activity, like walking or jogging in place, to get your blood flowing. Or, better yet, stretch *after* you exercise for maximum benefit.

Be cautious and always listen to your body when stretching – stretching a strained muscle can exacerbate the injury, so don't force it.

Stretching Tips

Stretch regularly

For maximum benefit, stretch at least two to three times a week after aerobic or strength training activity. Discontinuing stretching after having incorporated it into your weekly routine could decrease your range of motion and make it more difficult to participate in your other exercise activities. The goal of regular stretching, in addition to helping prevent injury, is to build up your flexibility over time, so stretching sporadically isn't nearly as beneficial.

Focus on major muscle groups

Stretch the major muscle groups in your arm and legs, as well as your lower back, neck, and shoulders. When you stretch one side of your body, make sure to stretch the other – left hamstring/right hamstring, right calf/left calf, left triceps/right triceps, for example. And pay extra attention to muscle groups you use often, tailoring them to your activity.

Aim for tension not pain

Tension means that your muscle is stretching, pain means you've gone too far and have pushed the muscle past a safe limit. If you overstretch, you can injure yourself, which means that you won't be able to participate in other exercises that involve the muscle you've injured.

Don't bounce

Some people think that bouncing the limb being stretched is beneficial, but it isn't. In fact, it's counterproductive. Bouncing during a stretch can cause little tears in the muscle, which leave behind scar tissue as they heal. This scar tissue actually renders the muscle even less flexible and leaves it more prone to pain. The key to good stretching is holding the stretch. Stretch until you feel tension (without pain) and hold the position for around 30 seconds without bouncing.

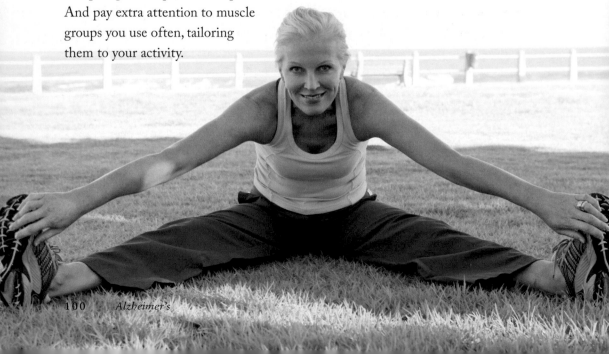

No Excuses!
Overcoming Exercise Barriers

True, it is easier to keep doing what you're doing than to change your routine, but if you are serious about beginning and sticking to an exercise plan, you need to overcome the urge to make excuses. Remember that no one is keeping score or grading you on performance – you are doing this because you care about your present and future health and you want to maintain your quality of life for years to come.

EXCUSE 1 — I'M NOT AN ATHLETE/ I DON'T KNOW HOW TO EXCERCISE

You don't need prior experience to get moving, all you need is the desire. Walking is an exercise that almost anyone can do for fitness. Set a simple walking goal – taking a walk around your neighborhood, for example – and if that feels good, do it again. Then set a goal for yourself that you will take that walk two or three times a week. You'll see that your fitness level and confidence will improve quickly.

If you want to go to the gym but feel intimidated by the equipment, seek the help of a physical trainer whose job it is to educate gym patrons on the various aerobic and weight machines at their disposal.

If you prefer to exercise at home, rent or purchase a fitness DVD – you can stop, pause, and rewind as often as you need to. Many of the fitness experts in these videos offer special instructions for beginners on how to perform their exercise properly and on when to take a break during a routine to conserve energy until you build up endurance.

EXCUSE 2 — I DON'T HAVE TIME FOR EXCERCISE

Most of us have busy schedules full of work and family responsibilities, but we also have a responsibility to ourselves (and to our loved ones) to be healthy for as long as we can be. If your schedule doesn't allow you to get in a full workout in one shot, exercise intermittently throughout the day.

Take a ten-minute walk on your lunch break. Instead of using the elevator, climb the stairs. If you can, wake up a little earlier than your usual time to exercise before your shower. Short spurts of exercise have benefits too.

Plan ahead. Make exercise a priority in your day. Lay out your workout gear and equipment at bedtime the night before so that you're not scrambling to find it in the morning. And schedule workout time like you would any other important appointment so that you'll be less likely to skip it.

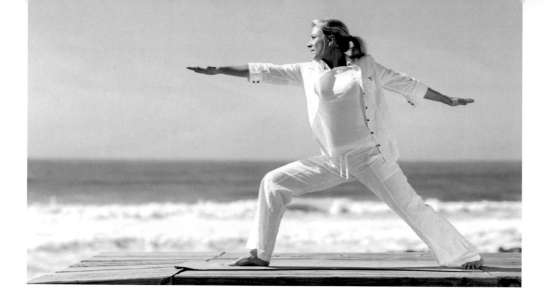

EXCUSE 3 · EXCERCISE DIDN'T WORK FOR ME IN THE PAST

Maybe you've tried exercising in the past and it didn't work out. That's ok, it's never too late to start over. If you decide to give exercise another shot, think about what made you quit in the past so that you can avoid it this time around.

Was it too grueling? Pace yourself. Don't set yourself up for failure with unrealistic expectations – realistically, you won't be able to walk ten miles on the treadmill or do 100 crunches on Day 1. Instead, start with a simple plan and build on it. Try walking once or twice a week, or following a tai chi video. Slowly increase your strength and stamina by setting and reaching small goals at your own pace, and eventually you'll see that you are capable of more than you thought you were.

Couldn't see the payoff? Don't expect results at once. Some of the benefits of exercise are invisible, like lower blood pressure and cholesterol, so you're making progress even if it appears otherwise. If you combine aerobic and strength training with a sensible diet, you will eventually see the results of your labor in the form of decreased body fat and increased muscle tone.

Were you too hard on yourself? You've made the decision to take care of your body and improve your health – there's absolutely nothing to feel bad about. If you are self-conscious about your appearance or your athletic ability, remember that where you begin today is a far cry from the results you will see in the future if you stick to your goals. Comparing yourself to other gym patrons or friends who have been exercising for a while will needlessly bring you down – when they started, they probably struggled too, but they stuck to their routine and saw the payoff. That will be you one day.

Tips for Staying Motivated

✔ **Do something fun.** Choose activities that you enjoy so that you'll be more likely to exercise.

✔ **Add variety.** Change up your routine too keep things interesting. Varying your workouts is good for your muscles too. Alternating the muscle groups you work out day to day gives muscles time to rest and repair.

✔ **Get a partner.** Working out with a friend is a great way to keep each other motivated. And you'll also be engaging in social activity – another protective factor for Alzheimer's disease.

✔ **Involve your family.** Schedule walks with your children or grandchildren. Play games with them in the park or swim with them at the local pool.

✔ **Join a health club.** Gyms offer a variety of fitness classes and equipment to choose from to keep you interested in exercise.

✔ **Schedule your exercise** during the time of day when you feel most energized. Some people feel at their peak when they wake up in the morning, while others have more energy in the afternoon. And if you need a pick-me-up, walking or jogging in place for 10 minutes will get your blood flowing and wake you up.

✔ **Remember why you started exercising** – you are on the path to better health and a better overall quality of life. Remind yourself that you are worth the effort it takes to keep moving every day.

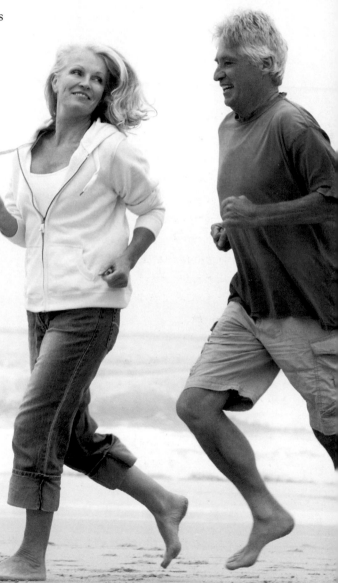

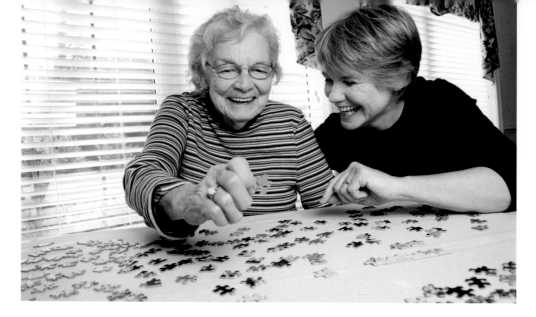

YOUR BRAIN – USE IT OR LOSE IT

Exercising Your Brain

As we age, our brain starts to shrink. As early as age 30 or 40, we begin to lose neurons that affect cognitive function. If the neuron loss is significant, it can lead to dementia.

The key to staving off these symptoms and regenerating neurons that make new connections in our brain is activity, both physical and mental. Recent studies show that aerobic activity increases grey matter, as does the act of learning.

Cognitive reserve refers to the mind's ability to resist or cope with damage to the brain. You begin to build cognitive reserve as a child, but the process continues as you age; therefore, you can build cognitive reserve at any time of life. When you exercise your brain, you increase your cognitive reserve and decrease your susceptibility to the symptoms of Alzheimer's and dementia.

The best way to maintain your brain power is to use it. If you find cognitively demanding activities that you enjoy, you will be more likely to do them regularly, and the less likely you will be to experience cognitive decline as you age. Activities that require focus, concentration, logic, and memory forge complex neural connections that the brain can call upon when pathways have been blocked by beta-amyloid and tau accumulation. These new connections can compensate for the ones damaged and destroyed by Alzheimer's. As such, people who actively seek out mental stimulation might have brain scans that reveal evidence of Alzheimer's disease pathology, but they might not experience the symptoms associated with it.

Using your brain every day – learning a new skill, studying a stimulating subject, playing challenging games and brain teasers, as well as engaging in positive social activity – help you build a bigger, more resilient brain. Keep your brain busy, well-rested, and stress-free, and you might postpone the symptoms of Alzheimer's indefinitely.

The mind has five main cognitive functions:

1. Memory
2. Attention
3. Language
4. Visual-spatial skills
5. Executive function
   (planning, organizing, remembering details, and managing time and space)

In order to stay mentally fit, try to incorporate activities into your life that address each of these functions.

Suggestions for Daily Brain Fitness to Delay the Onset of Memory Loss and Dementia

✔ Crossword puzzles
✔ Sudoku
✔ Ken-Ken
✔ Memory games
✔ Word search puzzles
✔ Reading
✔ Writing
✔ Language drills and word games
✔ Vocabulary building
✔ Attending lectures
✔ Playing an instrument
✔ Seeing a play
✔ Listening to classical music
✔ Assembling jigsaw puzzles
✔ Model building
✔ Quilting
✔ Online brain games and puzzles
✔ Brain games and training apps for your smartphone or tablet

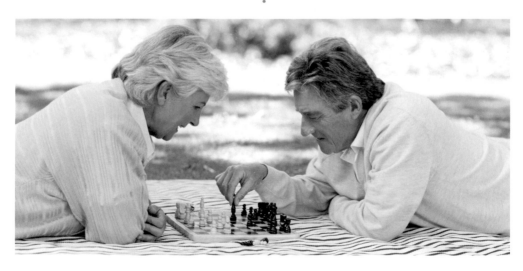

Lumosity - Online Brain Games and Brain Health

Lumosity is a brain training program that you can access on the Internet. Lumosity's brain training tools were developed by neuroscientists who have conducted extensive research in the field of neuroplasticity – referring to changes in neural pathways that can occur in the brain as an adaptive response to various injury or to learning. The creators of Lumosity assert that their program can improve cognitive function and increase cognitive reserve with regular use.

You can access Lumosity Mobile for your smartphone or tablet through the App Store (for Apple devices) and the Play Store (for Andriod devices.) You can also access the full Lumosity site through the Internet at **www.lumosity.com.**

The HAPPYneuron Method - Customized Online Brain Training

HAPPYneuron is a personalized and supervised online brain training method that can be tailored to suit your needs. HAPPYneuron uses games to stimulate the five main cognitive functions – memory, attention, language, visual-spatial skills, and executive function – increasing cognitive reserve and forging new neural pathways in the brain.

Each game lists the cognitive functions being exercised along with their benefit to daily life. Members can check a log of all their previous game results along with a list of achievements within the training and goals left to accomplish. The games adapt to your skill level as you improve, offering more challenging tasks and levels tailored to your past performance.

If you choose, you may take advantage of personalized coaching sessions to guide you through your training. Registration is free, and you may try out the program for a week, penalty-free before committing to purchase further sessions.

A series of apps exist for smartphone and tablet users – just search "happyneuron" in the App Store (for Apple) or in the Play Store (for Android.) The fully HAPPYneuron system can be accessed through **www.happyneuron.com.**

Lifelong Learning

Another way to build cognitive reserve is to commit to lifelong learning. Study after study has shown that people with more advanced educations are less susceptible to Alzheimer's than those who stopped their formal education at the high school level – the theory being that the longer you stayed in school, the better equipped your brain is to deal with the physical damage caused by Alzheimer's.

But don't worry if you never earned a Master's degree or went to law school. Learning can take place at any stage of life. Taking continuing education courses in subjects than interest you or acquiring

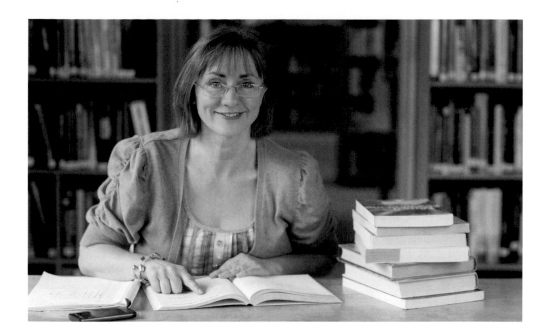

new skills can produce some of the same benefits as an advanced formal education.

Plasticity

Plasticity refers to the brain's adaptability when taking on new information. It was once thought that the brain was plastic only in one's youth – only children and teens can learn a new language or how to play a musical instrument, for example. But more recent theories on plasticity explain that a person can learn new skills at any age. The speed of acquisition might be slower, but lifelong learning is certainly possible.

You use the skills you already have to solve crossword or Sudoku puzzles – both good ways to stimulate the brain – but if you acquire new skills, you can forge even more complex neural pathways.

Anytime you learn something new, you are rewiring your brain, in other words, building cognitive reserve.

Learning facts in school – like the state capitals or the US Presidents, for example – is referred to as declarative learning. Declarative memory is language-based and analytical and involves the storage and recollection of facts that can be consciously stored in and retrieved from your brain.

Procedural memory, on the other hand, is typically acquired through repetition and practice. It is referred to as implicit learning, meaning that you know how to do something without necessarily being able to explain how. Procedural memory can be called upon without conscious thought and may have no language component. Consider how you ride a bike or tie your shoelaces. You most likely learned how to do these things decades ago, yet you still perform them today with little or no thought given to the process.

Challenge your brain by participating in lifelong learning that calls upon your declarative and procedural memory to build cognitive reserve. Age shouldn't be a factor in determining what you learn. The inherent plasticity of your brain will adapt to and thrive on the new information you acquire.

LIFELONG LEARNING SUGGESTIONS

✔ Take a continuing education course in a subject that interests you.

✔ Learn a new language.

✔ Learn new skills like woodworking or gardening.

✔ Learn to play an instrument.

✔ Learn new recipes.

✔ Take a dance class.

✔ Learn magic tricks.

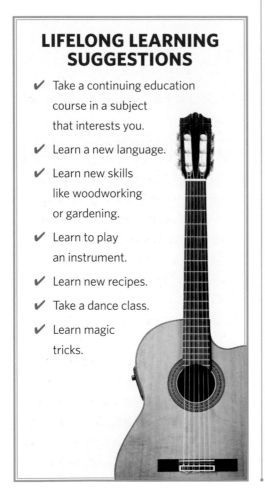

Sleep and Alzheimer's
The Restorative Power of Sleep

While exercise is essential for stimulating circulation and eliminating toxins from the body, sleep provides the deep rest necessary for the body to cleanse, repair, and rejuvenate itself on a cellular level. Much of the body's healing takes place while you sleep because it is not focusing on the other functions of daily life. During sleep, your body's immune system allows your liver and other detoxifying organs to process the chemicals and toxins that have built up during the day for elimination.

Even minimal sleep loss can take a toll on your mood, energy, and ability to handle stress throughout the day, and ignoring sleep problems can lead to poor health.

Sleep Takes Out the Trash

The precise reasons why our bodies need sleep largely remain a mystery; however, scientists have recently identified one reason our brains and bodies might work better after a good night's sleep. A team of researchers at the University of Rochester Medical Center in Rochester, New York published a study in the journal *Science* contending that waste is cleared more efficiently from the brain during sleep.

The study, which was conducted on mice, may lead to new ways to treat

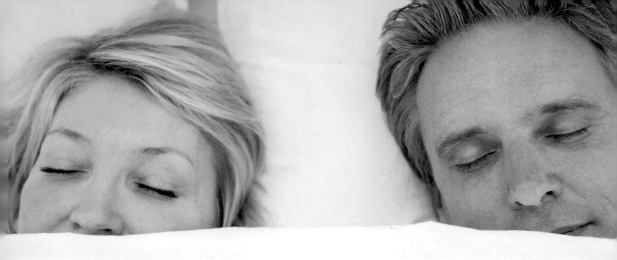

Alzheimer's and other brain disorders. Researchers discovered that beta-amyloid, which accumulates excessively in Alzheimer's patients, was cleared more rapidly from the brains of sleeping mice than from the mice that remained awake, reasoning that brain cells tend to shrink during sleep, widening the space between them and allowing waste to pass through.

To give your brain a fighting chance to remove Alzheimer's-causing waste, maintain a regular sleep schedule and get your sleep problems under control if you have any.

Handling Sleep Problems

Most people experience occasional sleeping problems, some of which can be improved without intervention from a doctor. The first step to overcoming a sleep problem is identifying and carefully tracking your symptoms and sleep patterns.

Keep a sleep diary A sleep diary is a useful tool for identifying daytime and nighttime habits that may be contributing to your sleep troubles. Your sleep diary will also prove a helpful reference if you eventually decide that you need help from a doctor or sleep clinic.

Your sleep diary should include:

✔ The time you wake up and go to bed each day
✔ Total hours of sleep
✔ Perceived quality of sleep
✔ Activities during your time in bed (times of sleeplessness, getting up to use the bathroom, going to the kitchen for warm milk, etc)
✔ The types and amounts foods and liquids you consume shortly before bed
✔ Your feelings and moods before bed (happy, sad, anxious, angry, etc)
✔ Any drugs or medications you are taking and the time of consumption

The more detailed you are able to be, the better. Your sleep diary might be able to help you to identify patterns that unlock the key to your sleep troubles.

Persistent sleep problems may be a sign of a more serious sleep disorder or an underlying medical condition such as insomnia, sleep apnea, restless leg syndrome, or narcolepsy.

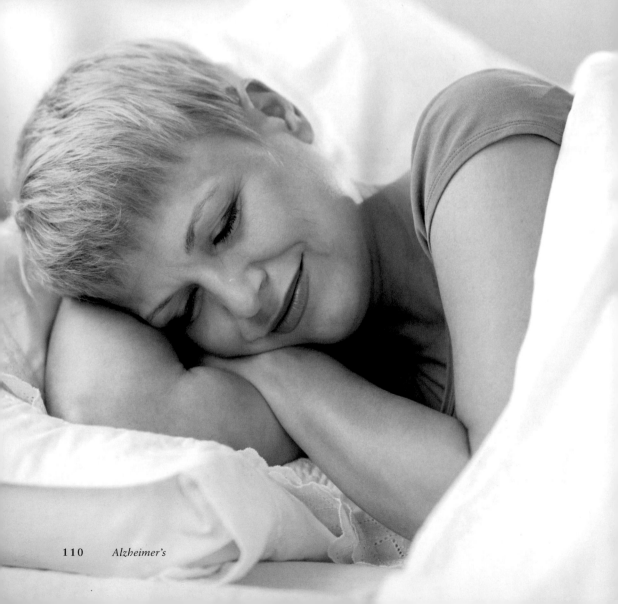

TIPS FOR BETTER SLEEP

Making simple changes to your daily routine could be all you need to do to get the sleep you need.

✔ **Keep a regular sleep schedule –** go to sleep and get up at the same time each day, including weekends.

✔ **Set aside enough time for sleep –** most people need at least 7-8 hours of sleep per night to feel energetic and productive during the day.

✔ **Create an ideal sleeping environment –** make sure your bedroom is dark, cool, and quiet. Use curtains or shades to block light from windows, and use a sleep mask if necessary.

✔ **Put away the electronic devices, including the TV –** the type of light smartphones, tablets and televisions emit can stimulate your brain, making it difficult to wind down and fall asleep. They also suppress the production of melatonin and interfere with your body's internal clock.

When to seek help

Persistent sleep problems may be a sign of a more serious sleep disorder or an underlying medical condition, such as insomnia, sleep apnea, restless leg syndrome, or narcolepsy. If making changes to your daily routine hasn't helped you sleep, it might be time to ask your doctor for advice or to visit a sleep clinic.

A specialist at a sleep clinic will observe your sleep patterns, brain waves, heart rate, and rapid eye movement. The specialist will then diagnose any disorders and design a treatment program based on your study results if necessary.

Signs you have a sleep disorder and need to see a specialist:

✔ You consistently feel irritable and sleepy during the day
✔ You have difficulty staying awake while sitting still, watching television, or reading
✔ You fall asleep at inappropriate times such as while driving, talking, or eating
✔ You have difficulty concentrating
✔ Others often tell you that you look tired
✔ Slow reaction time
✔ You can't control your emotions
✔ You need to nap almost daily
✔ You rely on caffeinated beverages or energy drinks to keep going

Overcoming Depression and Managing Stress

Depression

It was once believed that depression was a symptom of Alzheimer's onset. But more recently, studies conducted around the globe have shown depression to be a risk factor for the cognitive decline associated with Alzheimer's disease. Moreover, if a person withdraws from life due to depression, he or she is missing out on the kinds of mental activity and social engagement that are protective factors for the disease.

Maybe you feel blue from time to time when bad news comes your way. We all do – feeling sad after a major disappointment is a natural part of life. We may even say we're "depressed" in those instances, even though we are able to recover from the experience in a relatively rapid time frame.

But when feelings of sadness become so overwhelming that you cannot bounce back from them, and they interfere with your quality of life, you might be clinically depressed. Clinical depression can last for weeks, months, or even years and affects the way you feel, the way you think, and how you act. You might feel sad without being able to identify a reason, and you might withdraw from life, retreating from interests, activities, and people that were once important and enjoyable to you. Put plainly, you just don't feel like yourself anymore, and that feeling is not going away.

Common symptoms of depression include:

✔ Loss of interest in once enjoyable activities
✔ Withdrawal from friends and family
✔ An "empty" feeling
✔ Irritability
✔ Anxiousness
✔ Loss of appetite
✔ Feeling run down
✔ Trouble concentrating
✔ Crying for "no reason"
✔ Feelings of hopelessness
✔ Thoughts of suicide

If you think you might be clinically depressed, talk to someone about it. Seek help from a mental health professional like a clinical psychologist, licensed social worker, or marriage and family therapist who can diagnose your specific condition. Depression is highly treatable, and with the proper course of action, you could be feeling better in as soon as a matter of weeks.

Stress

Stress can limit the body's ability to detoxify. The body is made to handle stress in short spurts, not the week or month-long burdens of today. The connection between stress and our emotions can be a tremendous burden on the body. Chronic stress can affect blood sugar, disrupt sleep, and encourage bad habits like overeating and smoking.

STRESS MANAGEMENT TECHNIQUES

✔ **Have a workout.** Exercise is one of the cheapest and safest ways to combat stress. Exercise releases endorphins, which create a feeling of euphoria that can inspire a more positive outlook on life and ease tension.

✔ **Drink green tea.** Green tea contains the amino acid theanine, among whose benefits are helping to reduce psychological as well as physiological stress.

✔ **Breathe deeply.** Devote a few minutes of time to focusing on your breathing. Close your eyes, inhale deeply through your nose, hold your breath, and then exhale through your mouth, forcefully expelling all the air from your lungs. Repeat the cycle several times, inhaling, holding your breath, and exhaling for equal counts.

✔ **Practice meditation.** Meditation is a simple practice that can be done in a little as five minutes when needed. Sit in a comfortable position, close your eyes, and recite out loud or repeat in your mind a "mantra" or positive saying of your choice, such as "I am at peace" or "I feel relaxed." Don't try to force away distracting thoughts; acknowledge them and let them disappear on their own. You can find meditation guidance online or through apps on your mobile device.

✔ **Use a warm compress on your neck.** The warmth will allow your neck and shoulders to relax. When you remove the compress, ease away the tension with a hand massager or by rolling a tennis ball across the area.

✔ **Find ways to laugh.** Watch your favorite television comedy or film. Go to a comedy club, or chat with a friend with a good sense of humor. Laughing out loud lowers cortisol, a stress hormone, while increasing endorphins that elevate your mood.

✔ **Turn on your radio.** Listening to music has many health benefits, including lowering blood pressure, decreasing heart rate, and relieving anxiety.

✔ **Write it down.** Keep a journal or notebook handy to write down your thoughts. When you express a feeling in writing, you release it along with the associated tension it causes. Once you've expressed the negative thought, write down something positive happening in your life to counteract it.

Monitor the Quality of Your Information Intake

We are bombarded daily with disheartening news of war, economic setbacks, and tragic crimes, among other political and social upheaval – not to mention the bounty of celebrity gossip that dominates television, radio, and the blogosphere. With this ever-present barrage of news, we feel pressure to keep up, stay informed and on trend, lest we fall behind and get left out of the loop.

But the reality is that all of this news causes us much stress and anxiety with very little payoff in our daily lives. Focusing on bad news over which we have little to no control or on trivial celebrity gossip with no inherent value is a passive activity that does not stimulate our brains in a positive, beneficial way. In fact, this kind of information overload can have a negative impact on our disposition, mood, and self-esteem.

Be selective with your information intake. If you like to read the daily paper, do it – reading is a great way to stimulate your brain – but be sure to monitor the content of what you read. If you are interested in a particular topic or current event, read well-written, reputable content on the subject. Take care to limit the number of topics you focus on in a day, and try not to be distracted by endless news cycles that are manufactured to hold our attention without providing us with relevant, useful news.

Try taking a news fast – or at the very least, going on a news diet of one hour of news per day. Take the time you gain to focus your energy on gathering the kind of information that will positively impact your life. Learn how to plant a vegetable garden, read maps and historical texts on a place you plan to visit, or study a piece of sheet music you've been planning to learn – whatever topic interests you that adds value to your day. Your brain will respond positively to the pleasure of these activities and will benefit from the lack of stress that "news" can bring.

Social Activity

Social activity is a way to make physical and mental activity more enjoyable, with the added benefit of reducing stress, which helps maintain healthy connections among brain cells. Among people who have similar amounts of plaques and tangles in their brain, research has shown that those with larger social networks have fewer cognitive setbacks than people who are more isolated.

Staying Social While Keeping Fit

Combine social activity with physical activity for a one-two punch. Team sports and group exercise activate parts of the brain devoted to social interaction – so you're getting the dual benefit of physical fitness and mental stimulation with a single activity. Not only will you benefit psychologically from the interaction, but you and your friends can encourage each other as you exercise.

■ **Learn ballroom dancing**: A study published in the *New England Journal of Medicine* that was led by Albert Einstein College of Medicine in New York and funded by the National Institute on Aging revealed that frequent dancing is a protective factor for Alzheimer's. In addition to its cardiovascular benefits and social aspect, learning new dance steps enhances cognitive reserve by forcing the brain to carve out new neural paths, creating a more complex network of synapses for neurotransmitters to travel.

- **Buddy Up**: Make a regular golf date with a friend or play some doubles tennis. Any sport that gets you moving and provides intervals for socializing will work. Having an exercise partner at the gym is another great way to stay motivated. When you team up, you can help each other keep track of your progress, encourage each other through difficult exercises, and make each other feel more comfortable during a new exercise class. Plus, a little friendly competition between the two of you can push you to try a little harder to meet your goals.

- **Form a walking group**: Get a regular walking group together. It can consist of walkers from your neighborhood, or coworkers who all like to walk during lunch break, or members of any community to which you belong who are interested in improving their physical fitness. As long as you practice proper technique, walking and talking is a great way to pass the time while barely feeling the impact of your workout.

- **Play a team sport**: Join a team that plays in a league with a regular schedule like your local amateur basketball association, office softball team, or local bowling league. The camaraderie you form by playing together and working as a unit to win has immeasurable emotional benefits in addition to the physical.

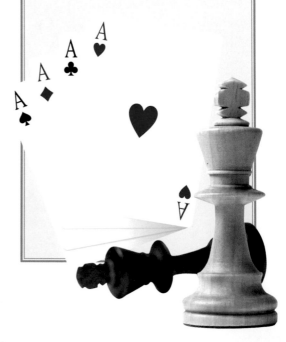

SOCIAL ACTIVITIES THAT KEEP THE MIND AGILE

✔ Playing chess

✔ Playing cards

✔ Playing board games

✔ Bingo night

✔ Book club

✔ Hobby clubs – puzzles, model building, photography, historical trivia, stamp collecting, etc.

✔ Taking historic tours

✔ Educational travel

✔ Museum tours

✔ Cooking class or cooking club

✔ Volunteering

✔ Having a pen pal (or email pal)

✔ Visiting family and friends

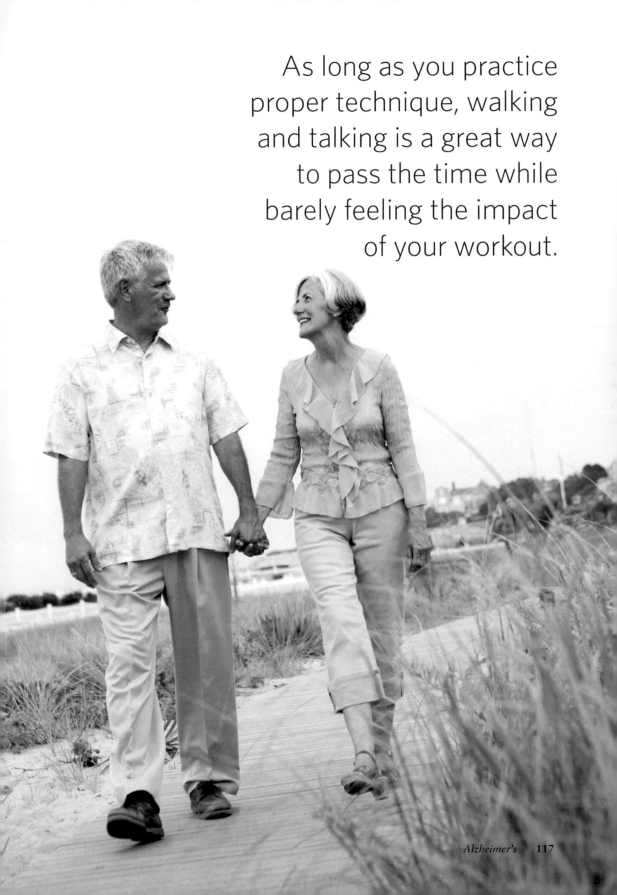

As long as you practice proper technique, walking and talking is a great way to pass the time while barely feeling the impact of your workout.

ALZHEIMER'S MYTHS

Alzheimer's only affects people's memory.

Memory problems are only one aspect of dementia. Other dementia symptoms include problems with speech and language usage, difficulties with spatial orientation, moodiness, and withdrawal. In the later stages of Alzheimer's disease, patients begin to experience serious physical complications as well.

If someone has dementia, it means they have Alzheimer's.

Alzheimer's disease and dementia are not synonyms. Dementia is a syndrome that is the primary characteristic of Alzheimer's disease. In fact, there are as many as 50 known causes of dementia including stroke, vitamin deficiency, substance abuse, head injury and brain tumors, in addition to Alzheimer's. It is crucial not to self-diagnose. If you suspect dementia symptoms, schedule an appointment with your physician to determine its cause so that you can receive the appropriate medically supervised treatment.

No one in my family tree has Alzheimer's, so I shouldn't be concerned.

The inherited form of Alzheimer's disease is very rare. Most people who have been diagnosed with Alzheimer's don't necessarily have a family history of the disease or a genetic predisposition. There are actually many risk factors beyond genetics that increase your likelihood for Alzheimer's.

I can get tested to see if I will develop Alzheimer's disease.

There are currently no screening tests for Alzheimer's available to the general public, although researchers worldwide are working to develop them. A test to screen for $APOE_4$ is only available for research purposes and is not administered for purposes of diagnosis because there is no corresponding therapy offered to address it. Instead, you can opt to participate in a research study that might offer you access to memory testing and top doctors at no charge.

Women have a higher rate of Alzheimer's disease simply because they outlive men.

While on average women do outlive men, researchers are exploring the role estrogen plays in post-menopausal women with Alzheimer's.

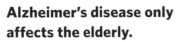

Alzheimer's disease only affects the elderly.

Alzheimer's predominantly affects older populations; however, people as young as 30, 40 or 50 can be affected. This is called early-onset Alzheimer's disease.

Current prescription medication can reverse the symptoms of Alzheimer's disease and dementia.

Currently approved prescription medication only temporarily relieves the symptoms of dementia in the early and middle stages of the disease for about 50% of patients. Nothing on the market today can either halt or reverse Alzheimer's disease, but scientists are working toward a cure.

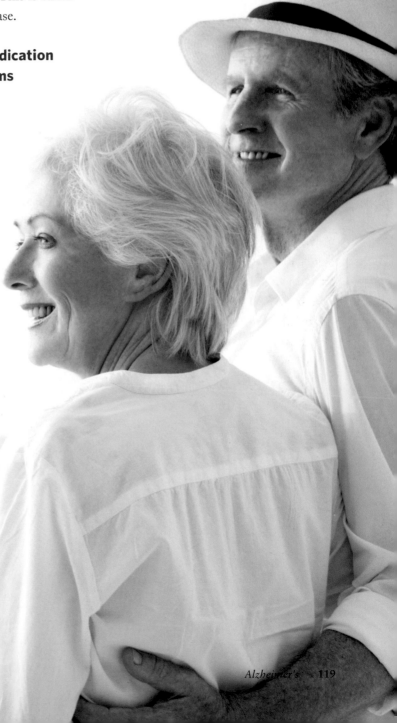

GLOSSARY

Acetylcholine: primary neurotransmitter involved with thought, learning, and memory; Alzheimer's may be linked to a lack of acetylcholine.

Acute: (of disease) brief and severe; acute inflammation occurs over seconds, minutes, hours, or days; opposed to chronic; acute inflammation is the cornerstone of the body's healing response.

Aerobic Exercise: an exercise that increases one's need for oxygen, thereby strengthening the heart and increasing blood supply to the brain; examples of aerobic exercise include walking, swimming, cycling, and jogging.

Amyloid Precursor Protein (APP): the precursor molecule that generates beta-amyloid.

Aphasia: the loss of a previously held ability to speak or understand spoken or written language due to disease or injury of the brain; aphasia is a primary symptom of advanced Alzheimer's disease.

Apolipoprotein E: the gene that produces protein that absorbs beta-amyloid and clears it from the brain.

Apraxia: a disorder of the central nervous system caused by damage to the brain and characterized by an impaired ability to carry out purposeful muscular movements; apraxia is a primary symptom of advanced Alzheimer's disease.

Asymptomatic: (of disease) without symptoms; the pre-clinical phase of Alzheimer's disease is asymptomatic.

Atrophy: (in Alzheimer's) the wasting away of the brain as a result of neural damage.

Beta-amyloid: (also amyloid beta, Abeta, or $A\beta$) a peptide of amino acids that is processed from the amyloid precursor protein (APP); the main component of amyloid plaques found in the brains of Alzheimer's patients.

Biomarker: short for biological marker; a distinct biochemical, genetic, or molecular characteristic or substance that is an indicator of a particular biological condition or process; blood and cerebrospinal fluid are examples of bodily substances being studied for Alzheimer's biomarkers.

Brain Stem: the part of the brain connected to the spinal cord and controls the body's automatic functions such as breathing, digestion, sense of touch, pressure sensation, and consciousness.

Cerebellum: the part of the brain that sits beneath the cerebrum and controls motor movement, coordination, balance, equilibrium, and muscle tone.

Cerebrospinal Fluid (CSF): the protective, clear, colorless fluid in the spaces inside and around the spinal cord and brain.

Cerebrum: the part of the brain that takes up the majority of the skull and controls memory, problem solving, intellectual function, emotion, and personality.

Chronic: (of disease) having a long duration; chronic inflammation occurs over months and years, causing rather than treating illness; opposed to acute inflammation.

Clinical Trial: a research study involving humans that rigorously tests the safety, side effects, and efficacy of a specific drug or behavioral treatment.

Cortex: the grey matter of the brain that covers the cerebrum (cerebral cortex) and cerebellum (cerebellar cortex).

CT Scan: short for computed tomography; imaging technique that uses x-ray equipment and computers to create cross-sectional images of the body.

Degenerative: a disease that becomes progressively worse.

Dementia: a syndrome whose symptoms result from damage to or loss of neurons in the brain; a state of serious mental and emotional deterioration; the primary characteristic of mild to moderate Alzheimer's disease.

Free-radicals: highly reactive atoms or groups of atoms formed in the human body that cause oxidative stress to cells, which then might malfunction and die.

Hippocampus: a part of the brain located under the cerebral cortex that plays a major role in short-term and long-term memory and spatial orientation.

Inflammation: the protective reaction of living tissue to injury or infection, characterized by heat, redness, swelling, and pain; inflammation is either acute or chronic.

Lumbar Puncture: the withdrawal of spinal fluid performed for the purpose of diagnosis; also referred to as spinal tap.

Metabolism: term used to describe all of the life-sustaining chemical processes in the body; metabolism is closely linked with the nutrition and essential nutrients that supply energy (calories) to the body.

MicroRNA: a genetic code fragment; microRNAs have been studied as possible biomarkers for Alzheimer's disease.

Mild Cognitive Impairment (MCI): a condition in which a person has memory problems greater than expected for his or her age but not on the level of dementia.

MRI: short for magnetic resonance imaging; imaging technique that uses magnetic fields to generate a computer image of internal structures in the body.

Nerve Growth Factor (NGF): protein important to the growth, maintenance, and survival of neurons.

Neural: of or pertaining to a nerve or the nervous system.

Neuron: a nerve cell.

Neurotransmitter: a chemical that delivers signals between neurons.

Nonaerobic Exercise: physical activity involving sudden, rapid motions, such as tennis, golf, or weightlifting that increases coordination, strength and flexibility but does not necessarily improve the respiratory and cardiovascular systems.

Oxidative Stress: damage caused to cells by free-radicals and can result in disease.

PET Scan: short for positron emission tomography; imaging technique that allows researchers to observe and measure activity in different parts of the brain by monitoring blood flow and concentrations of substances such as oxygen and glucose.

Plaque: amyloid plaque; insoluble deposits found outside neurons formed by excess beta-amyloid.

Synapse: the gap between neurons that allows neurotransmitters to pass between them.

Syndrome: a group of symptoms that are characteristic of a specific disorder; dementia is a syndrome characteristic of Alzheimer's disease.

Tangle: neurofibrillary tangle; a collection of twisted tau protein found inside neurons.

Tau: a protein found in the brain that, when abnormal, causes neurofibrillary tangles.

Vascular Dementia: dementia that develops after a series of strokes.

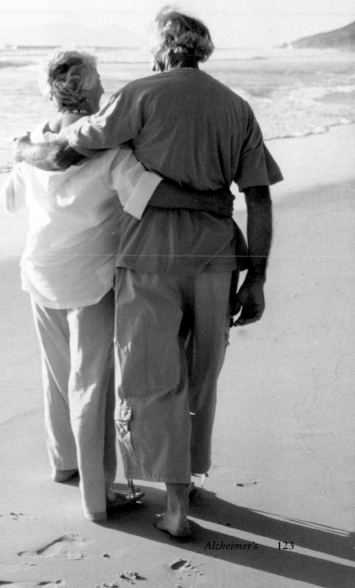

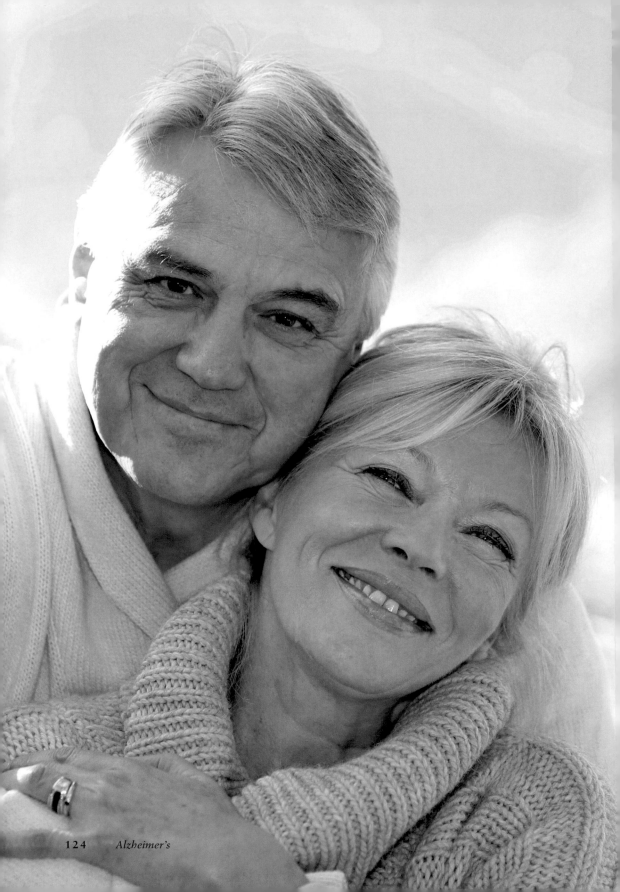

CONTACT INFORMATION

North and South America

United States

Alzheimer's Association
225 N Michigan Avenue
Suite 17004
Chicago, Il 60601-7633
Tel: +1 312 335 8700
Helpline: +1 800 272 3900
www.alz.org

Alzheimer's Disease Cooperative Study
University of California, San Diego
9500 Gilman Drive M/C 0949
La Jolla, CA 92093-0949
Tel: +1 858 622 5880
www.adcs.org

Alzheimer's Disease Education and Referral Center (ADEAR)
P.O. Box 8250
Silver Spring, MD 20907-8250
Tel: +1 800 438 4380
www.nia.nih.gov/alzheimers

Alzheimer's Foundation of America
322 8th Avenue
7th Floor
New York, NY 10001
Tel: +1 866 232 8484
www.alzfdn.org

National Institute of Neurological Disorders and Stroke
P.O. Box 5801
Bethesda, MD 20824, USA
www.ninds.nih.gov

Canada

Alzheimer Society of Canada
20 Eglinton Avenue, W.
Suite 1600
Toronto, Ontario M4R 1K8
Canada
Tel: +1 416 488 8772
Helpline: 1 800 616 8816
www.alzheimer.ca

Argentina

Asociación de Lucha contra el Mal de Alzheimer
Lacarra No 78
1407 Capital Federal, Buenos Aires
Argentina
Tel: +54 11 4671 1187
www.alma-alzheimer.org.ar

Brazil

FEBRAZ – Federação Brasileira de Associaçoes de Alzheimer
CF 542214 e o endereco
Rua Frei Caneca, 915
Conjunto 2, Sau Paulo, Brazil
Tel: +55 11 3237 0385
Helpline: 0 800 55 1906

Venezuela

Fundación Alzheimer de Venezuela

Calle El Limon, Qta Mi Muñe, El Cafetal

Caracas

Venezuela

Tel: +58 212 9859 183

www.alzheimer.org.ve

United Kingdom and Europe

Regional Group

Alzheimer Europe

145 route de Thionville

L-2611

Luxembourg

Tel: +352 29 79 70

www.alzheimer-europe.org

United Kingdom (except Scotland)

Alzheimer's Society

Devon House

58 St. Katharine's Way

London, E1W 1JX

United Kingdom

Tel: +44 20 7423 3500

Helpline: 0300 222 11 22

www.alzheimers.org.uk

Scotland

Alzheimer Scotland – Action on Dementia

22 Drumsheugh Gardens

Edinburgh

EH3 7RN

Scotland

Tel: +44 131 243 1453

www.alzscot.org

Belgium

Ligue Nationale Alzheimer Liga

Rue Brogniezstraat, 46

B – 1070

Brussel – Buxelles – Brussels

Helpline: (within Belgium) 0800 15 225

www.alzheimer-belgium.be

Germany

Deutsche Alzheimer Gesellschaft

Friedrichstr. 236

10969 Berlin

Germany

Tel: +49 30 315 057 33

Helpline: 01803 171 017

www.deutsche-alzheimer.de

Italy

Federazione Alzheimer Italia

Via Tomasso Marino 7

20121 Milano

Italy

Tel: +39 02 809 767

www.alzheimer.it

Netherlands

Alzheimer Nederland

Stationsplein 121

Post Bus 2077

3800 CD Amersfoort

Tel: +31 33 303 2502

www.alzheimer-nederland.nl

Spain

Confederación Española de Familiares de Enfermos de Alzheimer
C/ Pedro Miguel Alcatarena nº 3
31014 Pamplona (Navarra)
Spain
Tel: +34 902 174 517
www.ceafa.es

Switerland

Association Alzheimer Suisse
8 Rue des Pêcheurs
CH – 1400 Yverdon-les-Bains
Switzerland
Tel: +41 24 426 2000
www.alz.ch

Australia and Pacific

Australia
Alzheimer's Australia
P.O. Box 4019
Hawker, ACT 2614
Australia
Tel: +61 2 6254 4233
Helpline: 1 800 100 500
www.fightdementia.org.au

Hong Kong
Hong Kong Alzheimer's Disease Association
G/F, Wang Yip House
Wang Tau Hom Estate
Kowloon, Hong Kong SAR
China
Tel: +852 23 382 277
www.hkada.org.hk

Japan

Alzheimer's Association Japan
c/o Kyoto Social Welfare Hall
Horikawa-Marutamachi, Kamigyo-Ku
Kyoto
Japan 602-8143
Tel: +81 75 811 8195
www.alzheimer.or.jp

New Zealand

Alzheimers New Zealand
PO Box 14768
Kilbirnie
Wellington
New Zealand
Tel: +64 4 387 8264
www.alzheimers.org.nz

Singapore

Alzheimer's Disease Association
Blk 157 Lorong 1 Toa Payoh
#01-1195
Singapore 310157
Tel: 65 6353 8734
www.alz.org.sg

To locate your country's Alzheimer's association, visit **www.alz.co.uk**

INDEX